ELSEVIER'S
SURGICAL TECHNOLOGY EXAM REVIEW

ANBALAGAN GEORGE, MBBS, CST, MPE
Program Director
Surgical Technology
Eastwick College
Ramsey, New Jersey;
Surgical Technologist
Robert Wood Johnson Hospital
New Brunswick, New Jersey

JOSEPH E. CHARLEMAN, CST/CSFA, CRCST, LPN, MS
Program Chair
Surgical Technology and Sterile Processing
Berkeley College
Clifton, New Jersey;
Surgical Technician, Surgical First Assistant, and Operating Room Assistant Supervisor
Associated Surgeons of New Jersey
Englewood, New Jersey

ELSEVIER

ELSEVIER

3251 Riverport Lane
St. Louis, Missouri 63043

ELSEVIER'S SURGICAL TECHNOLOGY EXAM REVIEW   ISBN: 978-0-323-41493-7

Copyright © 2018 by Elsevier, Inc. All rights reserved.

Notices

Knowledge and best practice in this field are constantly changing. As new research and experience broaden our understanding, changes in research methods, professional practices, or medical treatment may become necessary.

Practitioners and researchers must always rely on their own experience and knowledge in evaluating and using any information, methods, compounds, or experiments described herein. In using such information or methods they should be mindful of their own safety and the safety of others, including parties for whom they have a professional responsibility.

With respect to any drug or pharmaceutical products identified, readers are advised to check the most current information provided (i) on procedures featured or (ii) by the manufacturer of each product to be administered, to verify the recommended dose or formula, the method and duration of administration, and contraindications. It is the responsibility of practitioners, relying on their own experience and knowledge of their patients, to make diagnoses, to determine dosages and the best treatment for each individual patient, and to take all appropriate safety precautions.

To the fullest extent of the law, neither the Publisher nor the authors, contributors, or editors, assume any liability for any injury and/or damage to persons or property as a matter of products liability, negligence or otherwise, or from any use or operation of any methods, products, instructions, or ideas contained in the material herein.

Library of Congress Cataloging-in-Publication Data

Names: George, Anbalagan, author. | Charleman, Joseph, author.
Title: Elsevier's surgical technology exam review / Anbalagan George, Joseph Charleman.
Other titles: Surgical technology exam review
Description: St. Louis, Missouri : Elsevier, [2018] | Includes index.
Identifiers: LCCN 2016042689 | ISBN 9780323414937 (pbk. : alk. paper)
Subjects: | MESH: Surgical Procedures, Operative--methods | Operating Room Technicians |
Perioperative Nursing--methods | Examination Questions | Outlines
Classification: LCC RD37.2 | NLM WO 18.2 | DDC 617.0076--dc23 LC
record available at https://lccn.loc.gov/2016042689

Senior Content Strategist: Nancy O'Brien
Content Development Manager: Luke Held
Content Development Specialist: Kelly Skelton
Publishing Services Manager: Jeff Patterson
Project Manager: Lisa A. P. Bushey
Book Designer: Ashley Miner

Printed in India

Last digit is the print number: 9   8   7   6

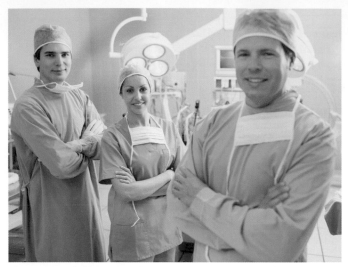

(Copyright © Wavebreakmedia Ltd/Wavebreak Media/Getty Images.)

WHY THIS BOOK?

This text is designed to help students, surgical technologists, and military personnel build content knowledge and develop study and test-taking skills in preparation for the two national certification examinations in surgical technology. In this introduction, you'll learn about the two exams—who gives them, the content areas they cover, how they're administered—plus how to prepare yourself to sit an examination and what you'll need to do on the big day.

THE EXAMS

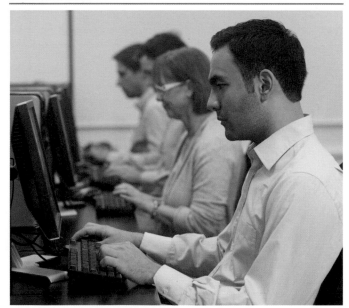

(Copyright © Wavebreakmedia Ltd/Wavebreak Media/Getty Images.)

As noted just now, two different entities offer certification examinations for those who seek credentialing as surgical

technologists: the National Board on Surgical Technology and Surgical Assisting (NBSTSA) and the National Center for Competency Testing (NCCT). Neither examination is universally accepted. It is your responsibility to research state laws, hospital requirements for employment, and the guidelines of pertinent healthcare organizations to ensure that you select the correct examination.

National Board on Surgical Technology and Surgical Assisting

Passing the exam offered by the National Board on Surgical Technology and Surgical Assisting (NBSTSA) allows you to use the title Certified Surgical Technologist, or CST. Graduation from a program accredited by the Commission on Accreditation of Allied Health Education Programs (CAAHEP) or the Accrediting Bureau of Health Education Schools (ABHES) is required of any student who seeks to sit this examination.

The NBSTSA exam consists of 200 questions: Of these, 25 are unscored questions that do not count toward a grade. Candidates must achieve a 67% grade on the remaining 175 questions, answering 118 or more correctly, to pass and obtain the CST certification.

The NBSTSA exam covers these content areas:

Preoperative care: 29 questions
Intraoperative care: 66 questions
Postoperative care: 10 questions
Administrative and personnel issues: 10 questions
Equipment sterilization and maintenance: 10 questions
Anatomy and physiology: 30 questions
Microbiology: 10 questions
Pharmacology: 10 questions
TOTAL: 175 questions

Candidates are allowed 4 hours to complete the test.

The NBSTSA provides exam outlines, test handbooks, and other exam resources to candidates. Use the following contact information to learn about the application process, obtain the exam content outline, find information on fees, and get answers to other questions:

NBSTSA
6 West Dry Creek, Suite 100
Littleton, CO 80120-8031
Phone: 800-707-0057
Fax: 719-328-0801
www.nbstsa.org

National Center for Competency Testing

The second examination that a candidate may sit to obtain surgical technology certification is offered by the National Center for Competency Testing (NCCT). Passing this test allows the candidate to use the title Tech in Surgery Certified (TS-C).

To take this examination, you must fulfill one of these qualifications:

- Be a current student in an NCCT-sanctioned school
- Be a graduate of an NCCT-approved school in the last 5 years

- Have accrued 3 years of full-time experience in surgical technology in the past 5 years
- Completed training in surgical technology, or an equivalent field, during U.S. military service in the past 5 years

Be sure to check the NCCT website for more specific information on these qualifications.

The NCCT exam covers these content areas:

Presurgical care and preparation: 44 questions

Intraoperative care: 70 questions

Postoperative care: 21 questions

Administrative and personnel: 14 questions

Equipment sterilization and maintenance: 26 questions

TOTAL: 175 questions

The NCCT exam comprises 175 questions. Test-takers are given 4 hours to complete the exam. Candidates must achieve a 70% grade to pass and obtain the TS-C certification.

The NCCT provides an outline of the examination, a candidate handbook, and other exam resources to all candidates. The application process, the outline, and the exam fees can be found at NCCTINC.com. Here's how to contact the NCCT:

NCCT

707 College Boulevard, Suite 385

Overland Park, KS 66211

800-875-4404

913-498-1243

www.ncctinc.com

Remember: It is your responsibility as a prospective test-taker to research diligently to ensure that you are preparing for the examination that best fits your needs.

EXAM PREPARATION

To get the best possible score on your examination, you must prepare properly. Let's discuss a range of strategies that candidates can use to ensure readiness for these certification exams.

- Time management
- Mindfulness
- Study tips and test-taking strategies
- Exam simulation
- Mapping

Time Management

Time management is essential in achieving a positive result on a competency-based examination. The candidate must schedule enough time for study and simulation before the exam. We all have busy lives, juggling work, family, education and other activities and demands on our time, so scheduling adequate study time will require you to evaluate your current schedule and priorities.

How much preparation time is enough? The candidate should be ready to study for no less than 12 weeks before the test date, dedicating at least 6 quality hours each week to studying and taking mock examinations, for a minimum of 72 hours of quality test preparation. The candidate should plan on two 3-hour sessions per week without interruption or disturbances. These sessions should take place outside the home—perhaps at the library, in a study hall, or any place where it will be possible to be alone to work without interruption. (Look for free Wi-Fi!) When disruptions arise, you will need to redirect your focus toward your goal of a successful exam and evaluate the threat to your schedule.

Table I.1 offers a sample study schedule for an exam candidate with work and family obligations:

You must create a realistic schedule that will fit into your life and *put it in writing*: This will help you commit to the schedule and make you more likely to follow it. Only you know where the holes in your schedule lie and where it will be possible for you to make the time to prepare for the examination.

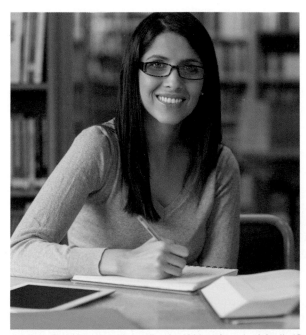

(Copyright © Wavebreakmedia Ltd/Wavebreak Media/Getty Images.)

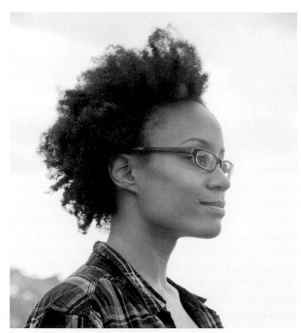

(Copyright © Nicolas McComber/E+/Getty Images.)

TABLE I.1   Sample Study Schedule

Time	Monday	Tuesday	Wednesday	Thursday	Friday	Saturday	Sunday
7 am–3 pm	Work	Work	Work	Work	Work	Family time	Family time
3–6 pm	Pick up kids; school activities	Pick up kids; school activities	Pick up kids; school activities	Pick up kids; school activities	Pick up kids; school activities	**Study for exam**	Family time
6–8 pm	Dinner	Dinner	Dinner	Dinner	Dinner	Dinner	Dinner
8–11 pm	Prepare for next day	Prepare for next day	**Study for exam**	Prepare for next day	Prepare for next day	Rest	Prepare for next day
11 pm–?	Rest and sleep	Rest and sleep	Rest and sleep	Rest and sleep	Rest and sleep	Rest and sleep	Rest and sleep

Mindfulness

Perhaps you've already heard the term *mindfulness*, a concept that has recently been getting a lot of attention in popular culture. Mindfulness is a theory that has been described in many ways by many psychologists, but they all boil down to this: succeeding by redirecting your mind, focusing on the present, and believing in your abilities.

The first step in cultivating mindfulness is evaluating your past experiences, because every decision we make is based on them. Redirect your attention to the present and away from the past. Take, for example, a student who has had a bad experience on an exam. Anxiety resulting from this experience will likely interfere with the student's preparation for the next exam. The candidate must clear the mind of all negative influences and pressures and instead focus on the goal of certification.

Finally, the candidate must believe that he or she can meet the challenge of a certification exam. Perhaps President Abraham Lincoln said it best: "Always bear in mind that your own resolution to succeed is more important than any other."

Perhaps you're thinking, "But what about my nerves?" It's OK to be nervous before an exam. Embrace your nerves and use the adrenaline they produce to stay alert and focused, but don't let them cancel out your preparedness or your intelligence. Perhaps you've had the experience of having to take a driving test as an adult because you've moved to a new state or let your license lapse. The thought of parallel parking for the examinee can be nerve-racking even if you've been driving for 20 years! But preparing for that driving test means that even though you're nervous, you're ready for the challenge.

Test-Taking Strategies and Simulation

To be successful on the actual certification exam, the candidate must prepare by creating the *experience* of the exam. Taking mock exams bolsters confidence by helping students become comfortable with the exam and what it will demand of them. Access to computer-based simulation exams is important for the candidate's confidence and comfort with the situation. Taking pencil-and-paper mock exams in preparation for a computer-based exam can have a negative effect on the candidate's score. Mock exams should be as close to the real situation as possible in terms of formatting, number of questions, and time restrictions. Students should make at least six simulation attempts before taking the actual certification exam. The example discussed holds true here as well: The more time a candidate for a driving test spends behind the wheel and practicing parallel parking, the better the candidate will perform on the actual test.

Many educators have favorite test-taking strategies. These include the following:

Rule Out

All questions on both the NBSTSA and NCCT exams are multiple choice. In the "rule out" strategy, the candidate eliminates (rules out) answers that have no relevance to the question. For example, say that a multiple-choice question on OB/GYN surgical interventions is presented. Any answer related to orthopedics, vascular surgery, or other specialty surgical intervention should be eliminated from consideration.

Never Change Your Answer

Once you've chosen an answer, don't look at the question again; consider all answers final. Going back to the question again will only give you the chance to doubt yourself and likely change a correct answer to an incorrect one. One instructor has said, "Once you answer the question, it goes in the vault. You may not look at it or touch it again." This strategy does require discipline, however! There is no rule saying that a candidate must answer the questions in order. Skip difficult questions and come back to tackle them later.

What Is the Question Asking Me?

The person who created the test question is looking to elicit a specific response to a specific piece of knowledge within the test question. Examine the question carefully and try to determine what the question-writer is looking for.

Candidates must be flexible in dealing with test questions, ready to draw on everything they've learned in many different subject areas. Students often say, when challenged with mock test questions, "I have no idea." Redirect them to use the knowledge they have acquired not just in surgical technology but also in the areas of medical terminology, anatomy and physiology, microbiology, pathophysiology, and pharmacology to evaluate the question and possible answers.

Study Tips

Though it's important to ensure adequate study time, studying for endless hours is not as important as "studying smart." How is this achieved? In four steps:

Step 1

The student must learn to apply fundamental knowledge of basic science and surgical technology didactic theory to achieve the entry-level knowledge needed to pass the CST exam. Think of it in this way:

Basic science + Surgical technology didactic learning
= Critical thinking + X

$$X = \frac{\text{Critical thinking}}{(\text{Basic science} + \text{Surgical technology didactic} = \text{Knowledge})}$$

$$X = \frac{\text{Critical Thinking}}{\text{Knowledge}}$$

$$X = \textbf{Passing CST}$$

Step 2

Use the knowledge derived from surgical "mapping," which we'll discuss in just a minute, to derive the intellectual reasoning.

Step 3

Take a web-based practice test provided by your school or tutoring agency.

Step 4

Prepare yourself mentally and physically for exam day.

Mapping

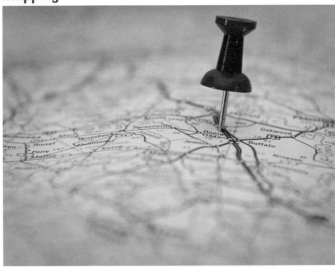

(Copyright © StockstudioX/E+/Getty Images.)

The key concept on which much of this book is based is **mapping**. In this system, we can take an organ in the body and (as a starting point) connect your knowledge of it (basic science + surgical technology didactic), then apply critical thinking.

As an example, let's talk about the **appendix**.

Basic Science

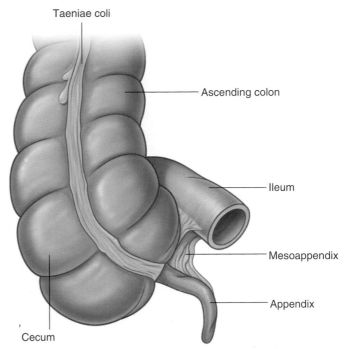

The appendix. (From Drake RL, Vogl AW, Mitchell AWM: Gray's anatomy for students, ed 3, Philadelphia, 2015, Churchill Livingstone.)

Medical Terminology

- The root word of the term *appendix*, *append*, is taken from the Latin word for "to attach."
- The suffix *-ix* means "pertaining to.

We'll talk more about how medical terms are built in Chapter 1: Medical Terminology.

Anatomy

- The appendix is a thin tube, about 4 inches long, that is attached to the intestines; hence, its name.
- Normally the appendix sits in the lower right abdomen, at the junction of the small and large intestines (the ileocecal junction).

Pathophysiology

What can go wrong with the appendix?

- Inflammation
- Rupture

Microbiology

Infection with certain bacteria can cause the appendix to become inflamed and eventually rupture.

- *Escherichia coli*
- *Klebsiella* species

Pharmacology

What medications are used in the surgical treatment of an inflamed appendix (*appendectomy*)?

- *Before surgery:* sedatives, IV fluids, antiemetic , antibiotic
- *During surgery:* anesthetic drugs, continuation of the IV fluids, muscle relaxants
- *After surgery:* reversal drugs, continuation of relevant medications

Surgical Didactics

Law and Ethics

What legal and ethical issues arise in the setting of a surgery like this one?

- Consent: written, verbal, and informed

Surgical Instruments

What instruments will the surgeon need to have sterilized and laid out properly for this procedure?

- General surgery minor set/tray
- The most important instrument, used in grasping the appendix: Babcock forceps

Procedural Steps

How is this procedure carried out?

- The patient is placed in the supine position
- After anesthesia is induced, a McBurney (right lower quadrant) incision is made.
- Muscle splitting is then performed.
- Once the appendix has been located and removed, a purse-string suture is used to close the stump of the appendix.

Wound Classification

What is the risk of infection during this surgery?

- Unruptured/inflamed appendix: class II: (clean contaminated)
- Ruptured appendix: class III (contaminated)

Possible Postoperative Complications

What could go wrong after the surgery?

- Hematoma
- Surgical site infection

Here you see the completed map for appendectomy:

SURGICAL MAPPING

Appendectomy (Muscle-Splitting Surgery)

Instruments	Important Anatomy Involved	Pathophysiology
General surgery minor instrumentation	Appendix Mesoappendix Cecum Ileum	Inflammation of appendix

Microbiology/ Wound Classification	Skin Prep/Incision/ Patient position	Pharmacology
Escherichia coli Class 2 (clean contaminated—unruptured appendix)	Midchest to midthigh McBurney incision Supine	Preoperative drugs Antibiotics Lidocaine/marcaine 50%/50%

Mapping Knowledge to Critical Thinking

Now that you've compiled the basic science and didactic knowledge of the appendix, it's time to apply some critical thinking!

We know the following information about the appendix:

- It is a hollow structure attached (root word *append-*) to the intestine.
- Its flora are similar to those of the cecum, to which the appendix is attached.
- Inflammation and the possibility of rupture are a common pathologic condition of the appendix.

- There is no significant loss of function if the appendix is removed.
- Removal of an appendix that is merely inflamed is wound class II (clean contaminated); removal of a burst appendix is wound class III (contaminated).

Here's where the critical thinking comes in.

An unruptured appendix represents a "clean contaminated" case. Why? Because the microorganisms are still contained in the appendix rather than moving freely in the abdomen. However, as soon the knife enters the hollow appendix, it is in contact with microorganisms, meaning that it (and all other instruments used to remove the appendix) becomes contaminated.

This knowledge takes you to the next step: how to continue with the surgical case management. As a means of preventing contamination, the appendix and all surgical instruments that come in contact with the specimen are deposited in a kidney basin, which serves as a neutral zone. Once the appropriate sutures have been applied and the wound is irrigated and closed, we can rest assured that this has been a safe and successful surgery and we've done everything possible to prevent surgical site infection.

No matter how much information you have about a situation, if you are unable to apply critical thinking to analyze it and respond appropriately, it will be of limited use to you. Keep this in mind as you make your way through this review.

CONCLUSION

We hope that this introduction has answered your questions about surgical technology certification exams, helped you devise a winning study strategy, and bolstered your confidence as you prepare to seek certification.

Now, on to our review!

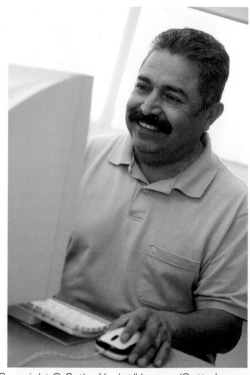

(Copyright © Cathy Yeulet/Hemera/Getty Images.)

CONTENTS

What's a Suffix?

A suffix is a word part that is added to the end of a root word to modify it or provide more information. Adding the suffix *–ology*, "the study of," to our example root word, *derm*, results in the term *dermatology*, "study of the skin." Table 1.2 shows some of the suffixes that are commonly used in health care.

What's a Combining Vowel?

Root words, prefixes, and suffixes don't always fit together in such a way that they're easy to pronounce. In these cases, a combining (or linking) vowel—often but not always /o/ or /a/—is used to help the word parts hang together a bit better. Take our example of the root word *derm*: Combining it with the suffix *–tologist* ("doctor of") results in the clunky *dermtologist*. Adding a combining vowel—*derm/a/tologist*—yields a much-easier-to-pronounce word.

Fig. 1.1 shows how a single medical root word can be modified to form many different terms.

Terms Not Based on Root Words

The other type of medical term encompasses terms derived from some characteristic—for instance, the person who "discovered" a disorder or structure or invented a tool or test, or some notable feature of a disorder. These names can't be broken into component parts and decoded; instead, they require simple memorization.

Names of Individuals

One well-known medical example of an eponymous (named after a person) disorder is Graves disease, an autoimmune condition of the thyroid. Robert James Graves published the first medical journal description of exophthalmic goiter, and the disorder is now named for him.

Descriptive Names

Many diseases, disorders, and injuries are named for their characteristics: how they appear (e.g., greenstick fracture, in which a bone is bent but not completely broken); where they're common (e.g., West Nile disease, first seen in Uganda); how they occur (e.g., stress fracture, caused by strain on a bone); who is subject to them (e.g., chimney sweep's carcinoma, a cancer of the scrotum caused by soot).

TERMS FOR BODY PARTS

Those of you who take the NBSTSA examination will be tested on body systems, so it is imperative that you know the names of the various parts of the body. Table 1.3 provides a sampling of terms for structures in each of the body's systems.

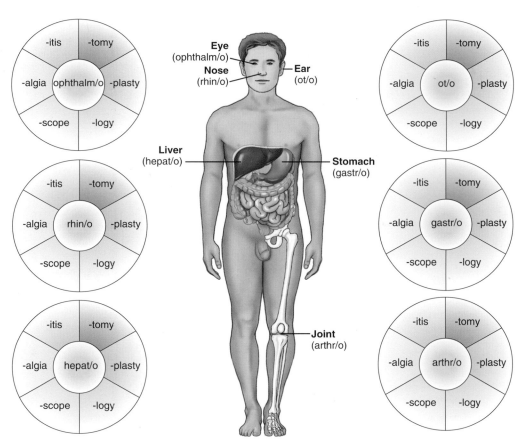

FIG. 1.1 Body parts and their combining forms. (From Shiland BJ: *Mastering healthcare terminology*, ed 5, 2016, St Louis, Mosby.)

TABLE 1.3   Body Parts, by System

Body System	Component Structures
Integumentary	Skin, nails, sweat glands, sebaceous glands
Digestive	Mouth, esophagus, stomach, small and large intestines, gallbladder, liver, pancreas
Genitourinary	Kidneys, ureter, bladder, urethra, prostate, testes, vas deferens, scrotum, vagina, uterus, vulva, ovaries, fallopian tubes
Cardiovascular	Heart, arteries, veins
Nervous	Brain, spinal cord, spinal nerves, cranial nerves
Respiratory	Nose, pharynx, larynx, trachea, bronchi, lungs
Skeletal	Bones, ligaments, tendons
Endocrine	Pancreas, pituitary gland, thyroid, parathyroid, thymus, adrenal gland, ovaries, testicles
Lymphatic	Lymph nodes

TABLE 1.4   Color Terms

Term	Meaning	Example
Cyan/	Blue	**Cyanosis**, a bluish discoloration of the skin, lips, or nails
Erythr/	Red	**Erythrocyte**, the scientific term for a red blood cell
Leuk/	White	**Leukocyte**, the scientific term for a white blood cell
Melan/	Black	**Melanoma**, a malignant tumor that often takes the form of a black skin lesion
Xanth/	Yellow	**Xanthosis**, an abnormal yellow coloration of the skin

COLOR TERMS

Several terms denoting color—which, by the way, is represented by the Greek-derived root word *chrom*–are used in medical terminology as both root words and prefixes (Table 1.4).

COMMONLY USED SURGICAL TERMS

Obviously, it's crucial for a surgical technologist to know the names of surgical procedures! Table 1.5 provides examples of the more frequently performed surgeries.

MEDICAL ABBREVIATIONS

Just as every profession has its own language, every profession also has its own shorthand—abbreviations and nicknames that make communication among members of the profession quicker and easier. Both for the sake of convenience and to help prevent potentially dangerous errors, it's a good idea to ensure that you're familiar with commonly used medical abbreviations (Table 1.6).

TABLE 1.5   Terms for Common Surgeries

Term	Definition
Abdominoplasty	Repair or modification of the abdomen for a more pleasing appearance (tummy tuck)
Acromioplasty	Repair of the acromion arch (shoulder)
Angioscopy	Endoscopic viewing of the heart and vessels
Angioplasty	Endoscopic repair of heart vessels
Anterior cervical diskectomy	Anterior approach to cervical disk removal
Anterior colporrhaphy	Cystocele repair, bladder)
Aortofemoral bypass	Bypass involving the aorta and femoral arteries
Appendectomy	Removal of the appendix
Arteriovenous fistula	Formation of a fistula between radial artery and cephalic vein for dialysis treatment
Arthroscopy	Endoscopic viewing of a joint
Arthroplasty	Repair of a joint
Bankart procedure	Repair of tear of labrum of glenoid capsule (shoulder)
Blepharoplasty	Surgery on eyelid to remove fatty or excess tissue
Bronchoscopy	Endoscopic viewing of the bronchus (unsterile procedure)
Carotid endarterectomy	Removal of plaque from the carotid artery
Carpal tunnel release	Procedure for neurolysis of median nerve entrapment
Cervical cerclage	Closure of an incompetent cervix
Cheiloplasty	Cleft lip repair
Chalazion	Small lump on the inner or outer surface of the eyelid
Cholangiography	Radiography of the common bile duct
Cholecystectomy	Removal of the gallbladder
Colectomy	Removal of the colon
Craniotomy	Creation of an opening in the cranium
Cranioplasty	Repair of a defect of the skull
Craniosynostosis repair	Repair (closure) of cranial sutures
Cystoscopy	Endoscopic viewing of the bladder
Epispadias repair	Repair of a congenital defect of the urethra on the dorsum of the penis
Embolectomy	Removal of an embolus (blood clot, fat, air, tumor) from the vascular system
Endometrial ablation	Removal or destruction of endometrial tissue
Enucleation	Excision of an eye duct to treat a malignancy
Entropion	Abnormal inversion of the lower eyelid margin
Gastrostomy	Creation of an opening into the stomach
Hysteroscopy	Endoscopic visualization of the uterus
Hydrocelectomy	Excision of the tunica vaginalis for removal of fluid
Hypospadias repair	Repair of a congenital defect of the urethra presenting on the ventral side of the penis
Illeal conduit	Urinary diversion from the bladder to a portion of the ileum
Ileostomy	Creation of a stoma from the ileum
Iridectomy	Surgical removal of the iris
Keratoplasty	Corneal transplant
Laparoscopy	Endoscopic viewing of the abdominal cavity
Lumbar laminectomy	Excision of lumbar lamina and removal of disk material
Mediastinoscopy	Endoscopic viewing of the mediastinum
Malar implants	Zygomatic (cheekbone) implants
Mammoplasty	Plastic surgery of the breast
Mastopexy	Breast lift by fixation of tissue

TABLE 1.5   Terms for Common Surgeries—cont'd

Term	Definition	Term	Definition
Mastectomy	Removal of the breast	Scleral buckle	Surgical repair of retinal detachment
Mastoidectomy	Excision of the mastoid process	Splenectomy	Removal of the spleen
Mentoplasty	Surgery to repair or improve the appearance of the chin	Strabismus correction	Repair of eye muscle to correct walleye or crosseye pathology
Myomectomy	Removal of benign fibroid tumors	Stapedectomy	Excision of otosclerosis of the stapes
Myringoplasty	Opening of the tympanic membrane	Subdural hematoma	Blood clot beneath the dura
Oopherectomy	Removal of ovary	Triple arthrodesis	Fusion of the subtalar, calcaneocuboid, and talonavicular joints (hindfoot)
Orchiopexy	Fixation of the testes within the scrotal sac		
Otoplasty	Ear repair	Thrombectomy	Removal of a clot that blocks blood flow
Palatoplasty	Cleft palate repair	Thyroidectomy	Removal of the thyroid gland
Pancreaticoduodenectomy	Partial or complete removal of the pancreas and duodenum	Tracheostomy	Creation of an opening in the trachea
		Transsphenoidal hypophy-sectomy	Procedure for removal of pituitary gland tumors through the upper gum margin (nonsterile) and into the cranium (sterile)
Parotidectomy	Excision of the parotid gland		
Phacoemulsification	Removal of an opaque lens by means of ultrasonic vibration		
		Tuboplasty	Repair of a fallopian tube
Pneumonectomy	Removal of a lung	Tympanoplasty	Repair of a tympanic membrane
Posterior colporrhaphy	Rectocele repair	Vena cava filter	Insertion of IVC filter to prevent pulmonary embolism
Prostatectomy	Removal of the prostate gland		
Pyelolithotomy	Excision of a calculus from the renal pelvis	Ventricular shunt	Placement of shunt to redirect cerebrospinal fluid from the cranial cavity to the peritoneum or right atrium
Rhinoplasty	Repair of a deviated septum		
Rhytidectomy	Facelift		
Rhizotomy	Surgical procedure to sever nerve roots	Vitrectomy	Removal of the vitreous humor from the eye
Salpingectomy	Removal of a fallopian tube	Vulvectomy	Excision and removal of the vulva

TABLE 1.6   Common Medical/Surgical Abbreviations

Abbreviation	Meaning	Abbreviation	Meaning
AAA	Abdominal aortic aneurysm	LAVH	Laparoscopically assisted vaginal hysterectomy
AC joint	Acromioclavicular joint	LEEP	Loop electrosurgical excision procedure
ACL	Anterior cruciate ligament	MMK	Marshall-Marchetti-Krantz procedure (urinary stress incontinence correction procedure)
AKA	Above-the-knee amputation		
A/P repair	Anterior and posterior repair	ORIF	Open reduction internal fixation
ASD	Atrial septal defect	PCL	Posterior cruciate ligament
BKA	Below-the-knee amputation	PDA	Patent ductus arteriosus
BSS	Balanced salt solution	PMMA	Polymethyl methacrylate (bone cement)
CABG	Coronary artery bypass graft	PNS	Peripheral nervous system
CHD	Coronary heart disease	POC	Products of conception
CNS	Central nervous system	SMR	Submucous resection
CSF	Cerebrospinal fluid	STSG	Split-thickness skin graft
C-ARM	A type of fluoroscope	T&A	Tonsillectomy and adenoidectomy
D&C	Dilation and curettage	TAH	Total abdominal hysterectomy
DCR	Dacryocystorhinostomy	TKA	Total knee arthroplasty
D&E	Dilation and evacuation	TMJ	Temporomandibular joint
DHS	Dynamic hip screw	TOF	Tetralogy of Fallot
DUB	Dysfunctional uterine bleeding	TRAM	Transverse rectus abdominis musculocutaneous flap
ECG	Electrocardiogram	TURBT	Transurethral resection of bladder tumor
EEG	Electroencephalograph	TURP	Transurethral resection of prostate
ESU	Electrosurgical unit	UA	Urinalysis
FESS	Functional endoscopic sinus surgery	UPPP	Uvulopalatopharyngoplasty
FTSG	Full-thickness skin graft	VAD	Ventricular assist device
HNP	Herniated nucleus pulposus	VATS	Video-assisted thoracic surgery
IABP	Intraaortic balloon pump	VSD	Ventricular septal defect

CONCLUSION

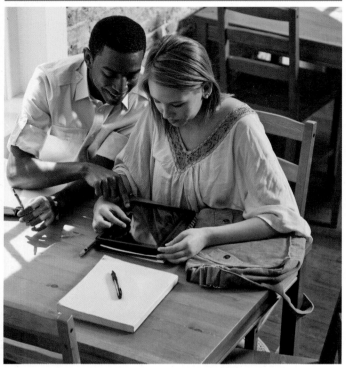

(Copyright © Susan Chiang/E+/Getty Images.)

In this chapter, we've touched on just a sampling of the thousands of medical terms in use today. You'll encounter still more as you make your way through this review text. If you feel ready, quiz yourself with the Review Questions. The answers are available on the Evolve Resources site, along with practice exam questions.

REVIEW QUESTIONS

1. Hysterectomy is surgical removal of the:
   a. Liver
   b. Uterus
   c. Ovaries
   d. Stomach
2. The suffix in the word neuralgia means:
   a. Cell
   b. Pain
   c. Nerve
   d. Strength
3. The prefix in the word *suprapubic* means:
   a. Below
   b. Above
   c. Perineal
   d. Enlarged
4. Which acronym refers to the open fixation of a fracture?
   a. ACL
   b. BSO
   c. TAH
   d. ORIF
5. The suffix of the word *osteoarthritis* refers to:
   a. Bone
   b. Joint
   c. Infection
   d. Inflammation
6. Diego, the CST on call, is told to prepare for an emergency gastrectomy. What kind of surgery is this?
   a. Repair of the esophagus
   b. Removal of the stomach
   c. Visualization of the intestines
   d. Creation of an opening into the stomach
7. The suffix in the word *cardiomegaly* means:
   a. Heart
   b. Muscle
   c. Enlarged
   d. Lacking tone
8. The prefix in the word *dysmenorrhea* means:
   a. Pain
   b. Flow
   c. Heavy
   d. Menses
9. The abbreviation *TAH /BSO* is short for "total abdominal hysterectomy and:
   a. Bilateral suturing of the os
   b. Bilateral stapling of the ovary
   c. Removal of the broad ligament
   d. Removal of the ovaries and fallopian tubes
10. Which suffix refers to death?
    a. -al
    b. -itis
    c. -necrosis
    d. -cyanosis
11. Which root word refers to cartilage?
    a. Oste/o
    b. Arthr/o
    c. Chondr/o
    d. Menisc/o

12. During a shoulder procedure, the surgeon asks the CST to place the patient's arm in adduction. What does the prefix of this word indicate that the surgeon wants?
    a. Away
    b. Below
    c. Above
    d. Toward
13. What part of the anatomy is affected by keratoplasty?
    a. Eye
    b. Ear
    c. Colon
    d. Kidney
14. On what part of the anatomy is myringotomy performed?
    a. Nose
    b. Tonsil
    c. Throat
    d. Eardrum
15. What does the suffix of the word *carcinoma* indicate?
    a. Tumor
    b. Benign
    c. Cancer
    d. Metastasis
16. A CST overhears a surgeon saying that they will be creating an opening into the patient's small intestine. What is the name of this procedure?
    a. Ileostomy
    b. Colectomy
    c. Colonoscopy
    d. Sigmoidoscopy
17. The suffix of the word *arthroscopy* refers to:
    a. Joint
    b. Repair
    c. Fusion
    d. Viewing
18. *Cryptorchidism* is the term for the condition in which a testicle is undescended. What is the name of the procedure used to fix this problem?
    a. Vasectomy
    b. Orchiopexy
    c. Orchiectomy
    d. Vasovasotomy
19. What does the suffix of the word *herniorrhaphy* mean?
    a. Fixation
    b. Suturing
    c. Repairing
    d. Weakness
20. What is the name of the surgical intervention needed for a patient who has sustained an injury to the ear?
    a. Otoplasty
    b. Rhinoplasty
    c. Rhytidectomy
    d. Blepharoplasty
21. What is the word for an increase in the size of an organ or structure?
    a. Hypotrophy
    b. Hypoplasia
    c. Hypertrophy
    d. Hyperaggressive
22. The name of the instrument used to cut an exostosis from a bone is:
    a. Ocutome
    b. Distractor
    c. Osteotome
    d. Arthroscope
23. Dead matter that is cast off from the skin's surface after a burn is called:
    a. Eschar
    b. Epidermis
    c. Dermatitis
    d. Subcutaneous
24. The surgeon worries that a particular kind of mass, which could be solid, gaseous, or liquid, will develop in a patient. What is the name of this mass?
    a. Tumor
    b. Embolus
    c. Thrombus
    d. Hematoma
25. Escape of fluid into an area or part is termed:
    a. Osmosis
    b. Effusion
    c. Diffusion
    d. Condensation

2

Anatomy and Physiology

OUTLINE—CONT'D

Anatomy and physiology, or A&P, are subjects that just about every student assumes will be among the most difficult to study. True, it requires a lot of memorization, and many people don't have the patience to study, tending to look for shortcuts and cheat sheets and so forth to pass their tests instead. Those of you considering the easy way out need to ask yourself this question: **Why is knowledge of anatomy and physiology important for the surgical technologist?**

Here's why: The surgical technologist, a member of an advanced allied health profession, *must* have a basic working knowledge of A&P to do the job safely and well. Knowing the parts and systems of the human body and how they work will help you understand and anticipate the steps of surgical procedures much more effectively.

We believe that studying A&P productively requires patience and consistency. There's no denying that this subject matter is complicated, but there are ways in which you can learn and retain the material— you just have to be **consistent**. This will help you become familiar with the subject, and familiarity fosters memorization and understanding.

One means of improving your understanding and recall is to **draw pictures** of what you're studying—or, if you're not an artist, just cut out pictures of the anatomy and stick them around your study room. Look at them every day. Trust me: our brains function just like a camera, and the more time you spend looking at the images, the more deeply they will be registered in your memory bank.

Complicated though it might be, anatomy and physiology is also *fun*. Here's just a tiny sampling of fascinating A&P facts:

- Let say you decide to try eating while standing on your head. Even upside down, the smooth muscle of the esophagus will continue to do its job, moving in a wavelike motion, until the food is deposited safely in your stomach. (It takes 2 to 5 seconds for food to travel from the mouth to the stomach.)
- Over a 24-hour period, the salivary glands will produce 1.7 L of fluid.
- In the average adult, 11.5 L of food, liquids, and digestive juices makes its way through the digestive system over the course of 24 hours, but only 100 mL is lost in feces.
- Your entire digestive system, from mouth to anus, is 30 feet long; the small intestine is about 22 feet (7 m) long.
- The hydrochloric acid found in our stomachs is the same substance used by masons to clean bricks.
- The human gastrointestinal system plays host to more than 500 species of bacteria.
- Intestinal gas, or flatus, is a combination of swallowed air and the gases produced by the fermentation of bacteria in the gastrointestinal tract. Certain components of food can't be broken down or absorbed by the digestive system, and those substances are simply pushed along the tract and into the large intestine (a.k.a. the colon). Hordes of intestinal bacteria in the colon go to work, releasing a variety of gases in the process, including carbon dioxide, hydrogen, methane, and hydrogen sulfide, which gives flatulence its rotten-egg stench.

PREPARING FOR A CERTIFICATION EXAM

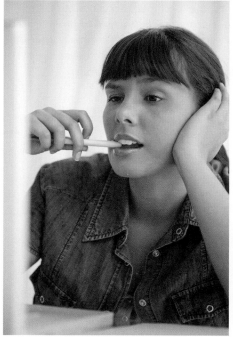

(Copyright © Wavebreakmedia Ltd/Wavebreak Media/Getty Images.)

Before we get started on our review, let's talk about what's going to be asked of you, in terms of anatomy and physiology, on your certification examination. Here are the expectations set forth in the outline provided by the NBSTSA.

- Use appropriate medical terminology and abbreviations.
- Demonstrate knowledge of these anatomical systems and their physiology **as they relate to the surgical procedure:**
  - Cardiovascular
  - Gastrointestinal
  - Endocrine
  - Integumentary
  - Lymphatic
  - Muscular
  - Neurological
  - Peripheral vascular
  - Reproductive
  - Pulmonary
  - Otorhinolaryngologic
  - Skeletal
  - Genitourinary
  - Ophthalmic
- Identify the following **surgical pathologies**:
  - Abnormal anatomy
  - Disease process
  - Traumatic injuries
  - Malignancies

In this chapter we'll be making our way through these lists to ensure that you can tie anatomy and physiology together in the context of pathologic conditions treated with surgery. Let's get to work!

CARDIOVASCULAR SYSTEM

CABG (Coronary Artery Bypass Graft)

See Fig. 2.1. What parts of the anatomy are affected by this procedure?
- Aorta (becomes occluded, necessitating CABG)
- Sternum (sternotomy performed to provide access)
- Coronary artery (subjected to coronary arteriotomy)
- Internal mammary artery (harvested as a graft)
- Saphenous vein (harvested as a graft)

Remember, the NBSTA exam will require you to know the surgical pathologies, which include abnormal anatomy, disease process, traumatic injuries, and malignancies, if any, related to the procedure or to find a better way to understand why the patient is scheduled for CABG.

Mapping

Remember the mapping method we discussed in the Introduction? Here's where we start using it. Let's map some commonly performed cardiovascular procedures.

SURGICAL MAPPING

CABS

Related Anatomy	Abnormal Anatomy	Pathology
Coronary artery	Blocked coronary artery	Arteriosclerosis (buildup of cholesterol deposits in the arterial lining)
Internal mammary artery		
Saphenous vein		Heart muscle weakening (ischemia) leading to myocardial infarction
Sternum		
Aorta		

Aortic Valve Replacement

What parts of the anatomy are affected by this procedure?
- Ascending aorta (becomes occluded)
- Aortic valve (requires replacement)
- Sternum (sternotomy performed to provide access)

Mapping

SURGICAL MAPPING

Aortic valve replacement

Related Anatomy	Abnormal Anatomy	Pathology
Sternum	Aortic valve:	Calcification
Ascending aorta	Prolapse	Congenital abnormalities
Aortic valve	Inability to close	
	Stenosis	Endocarditis

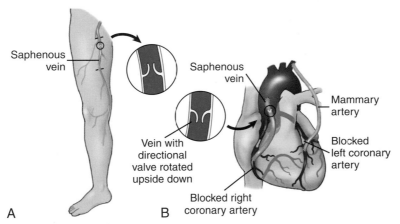

FIG. 2.1 Coronary artery bypass graft (CABG) surgery. (From Shiland BJ: Medical Terminology & Anatomy for ICD-10 Coding, ed 2, 2015, St Louis, Mosby.)

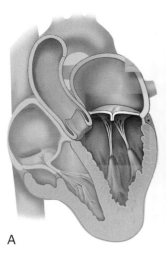
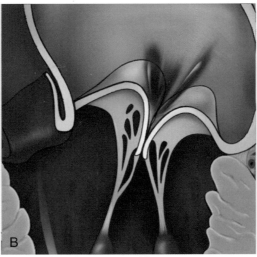
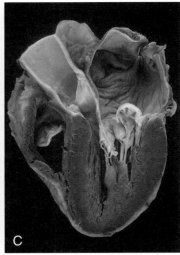

A   B   C

FIG. 2.2 Mitral valve prolapse. The normal mitral valve *(upper left)* prevents backflow of blood from the left ventricle into the left atrium during ventricular systole (contraction). The prolapsed mitral valve *(right)* permits leakage because the valve flaps billow backward, parting slightly. The photo inset shows the ballooning *(arrow)* of the mitral valve into the atrium. (Drawings from Patton KT, Thibodeau GA: The Human Body in Health and Disease, ed 6, 2014, St Louis, Mosby; photo courtesy of William D Edwards, MD, Mayo Clinic, Rochester, MN.)

Mitral Valve Replacement

See Fig. 2.2. What anatomy is affected by this procedure?
- Ascending aorta (becomes occluded)
- Mitral valve (a.k.a. bicuspid valve, between the left atrium and left ventricle)
- Sternum (sternotomy for the purpose of access)

Mapping

Let's map this aortic procedure:

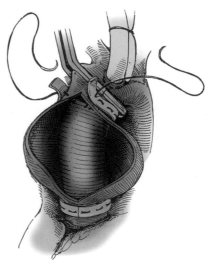

FIG. 2.3 Repair of aneurysm of ascending aorta. (From Waldhausen JA et al: Surgery of the chest, ed 6, St Louis, 1996, Mosby.)

SURGICAL MAPPING		
Mitral valve replacement		
Related Anatomy	**Abnormal Anatomy**	**Pathology**
Sternum	Mitral valve:	Rheumatic heart disease
Ascending aorta	Prolapse	Dilation of the annulus
Mitral valve	Inability to close	Ischemic heart disease
	Stenosis	Trauma
		Tissue changes that produce regurgitation

Resection of Aneurysm of the Ascending Aorta

See Fig. 2.3. What parts of the anatomy are affected by this procedure?
- Aorta
- Sternum (sternotomy performed to provide access)
- Aortic valve
- Femoral artery (used as a graft)
- Coronary arteries

Mapping

Here you can see how this procedure maps:

SURGICAL MAPPING		
Resection of aneurysm of the ascending aorta		
Related Anatomy	**Abnormal Anatomy**	**Pathology**
Sternum	Aortic wall balloons	Arteriosclerosis
Ascending aorta	out:	Atherosclerosis
Aortic valve	Saccular aneurysm	Delamination of the intimal
Coronary arteries	Fusiform aneurysm	layer of the aorta
Femoral artery		(dissecting aneurysm)

Recipient's heart during surgery

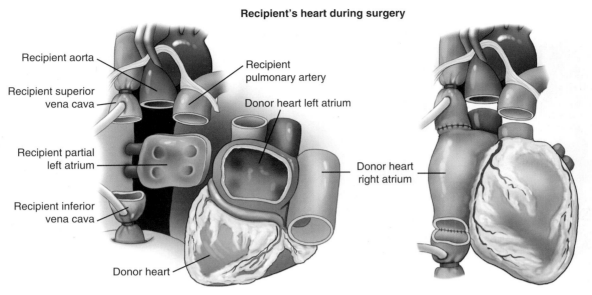

FIG. 2.4 Heart transplantation.

Heart Transplantation

See Fig. 2.4. What parts of the anatomy are affected by this procedure?

- Sternum (sternotomy performed to provide access)
- Pulmonary veins
- Pulmonary arteries
- Orthotopic heart

Mapping

Let's lay the procedure out in a map:

SURGICAL MAPPING

Heart Transplantation

Related Anatomy	Abnormal Anatomy	Pathology
Sternum	Failure of heart	Coronary artery disease
Pulmonary veins		Congenital heart disease
Pulmonary arteries		Valve disease
Orthotopic heart		Rejection of previously transplanted heart

Other Cardiovascular Procedures

Now it's your turn to do some mapping! Using the template provided on the Evolve Resources site, map out each procedure—name, related anatomy, abnormal anatomy, and pathology—for each of the following cardiac procedures.

- Cardiac pacemaker insertion
- Endovascular repair of thoracic aneurysm
- Pericardial window
- Insertion of a ventricular assist device (VAD)

GASTROINTESTINAL SYSTEM

The gastrointestinal system comprises much more than just the stomach and intestines (Fig. 2.5). Let's have a quick review of the areas and organs of the gastrointestinal tract before we start mapping the surgeries that affect them.

Divisions of the Abdomen
Quadrants

See Fig. 2.6.

- Right upper quadrant
- Right lower quadrant
- Left upper quadrant
- Left lower quadrant

Regions

See Fig. 2.7.

- Right hypochondrium
- Right lumbar region
- Right iliac fossa region
- Epigastrium
- Umbilical region
- Hypogastric or suprapubic region
- Left hypochondrium
- Left lumbar region
- Left iliac fossa region

Tissue Layers: Superficial to Deep

- Skin
- Subcutaneous fatty tissues
- Fascia
- Muscle
- Peritoneum

Organs of the Gastrointestinal System
Digestive Tract

These organs extract nutrients and water from food for the nourishment of the body and then get rid of any waste material remaining.

- Esophagus: smooth muscle–lined tube through which chewed food, liquids, and saliva travel from the mouth to the stomach by means of peristalsis
- Stomach: muscular pouch where food is exposed to secretions to aid digestion before being moved along to the small intestine

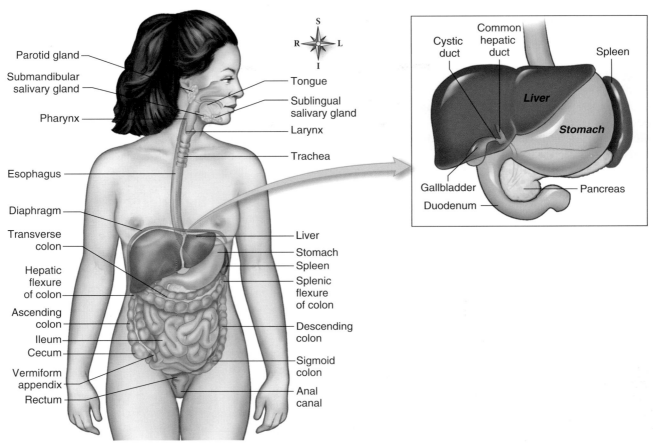

FIG. 2.5 Location of the digestive organs. (From Patton KT, Thibodeau GA: The Human Body in Health and Disease, ed 6, 2014, St Louis, Mosby.)

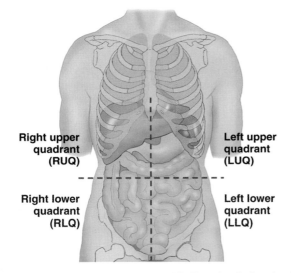

FIG. 2.6 Abdominal quadrants. (© Elsevier Collection.)

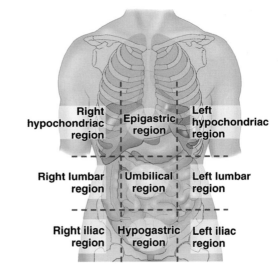

FIG. 2.7 Abdominopelvic regions. (© Elsevier Collection.)

- Small intestine: long tubular organ that receives partially digested food (chyme) from the stomach, as well as bile from the liver and digestive enzymes from the pancreas to further break down the food into nutrients
- Large intestine (a.k.a colon): a second long tubular organ; receives mostly digested food from the small intestine, extracts water from the digested food, and forms waste material into feces
- Rectum: final section of the large intestine, where feces are stored before expulsion
- Anus: muscular ring through which feces are expelled from the body; terminus of the digestive tract.

Accessory Digestive Organs

Liver. See Fig. 2.8. The liver has many responsibilities:
- Processing blood to remove nutrients, toxins, and medications
- Storing energy in the form of glycogen
- Storing vitamins and minerals and releasing them as the body needs them
- Producing proteins needed for blood clotting
- Producing bile, which aids digestion

Gallbladder. This structure stores the bile that the liver produces until it is needed for digestion.

Pancreas. This organ belongs to both the digestive and endocrine systems (Fig. 2.9).
- The pancreas contains structures known as the islets of Langerhans, made up of cells that secrete hormones:
  - Alpha cells secrete glucagon.
  - Beta cells secrete insulin.

- The pancreas also produces an enzyme that aids in digestion, as well as bicarbonate, which neutralizes stomach acid before it reaches the small intestine.

Spleen. See Fig. 2.10. Like the liver and pancreas, this organ does several jobs:
- It holds a reserve of blood to counteract hemorrhagic shock.
- It removes from circulation and destroys aged red blood cells.
- It makes antibodies to aid immune response.
- It stores half the body's monocytes, which differentiate into several cell types as needed.

Gastrointestinal Surgeries
Hernia Repair
A hernia is a protrusion of abdominal contents through a weakened area of the abdominal wall (Fig. 2.11).

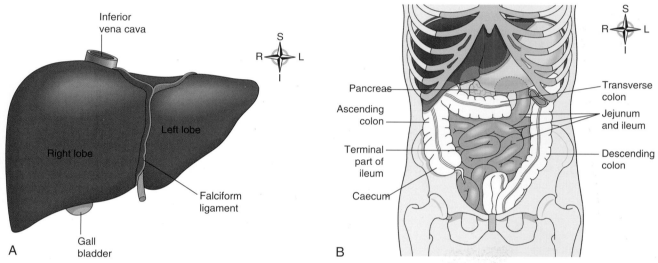

FIG. 2.8 The liver. **A,** anterior view. **B,** turned up to show posterior surface. (From Waugh A, Grant A: Ross and Wilson Anatomy & Physiology in Health and Illness, ed 12, Edinburgh, 2014, Churchill Livingstone.)

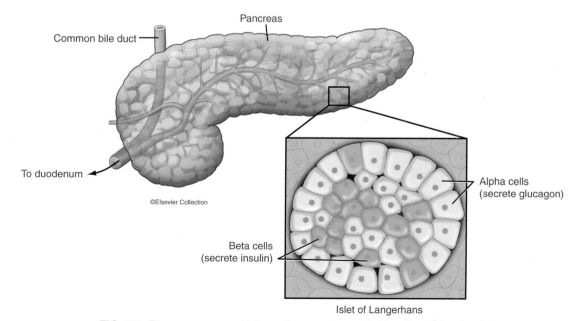

FIG. 2.9 The pancreas and islets of Langerhans. (© Elsevier Collection.)

What parts of the anatomy are affected by this procedure? That depends on the type of hernia.

- Omentum (most commonly)
- Small intestine

Mapping

Let's organize the pertinent information on hernia repair into a map:

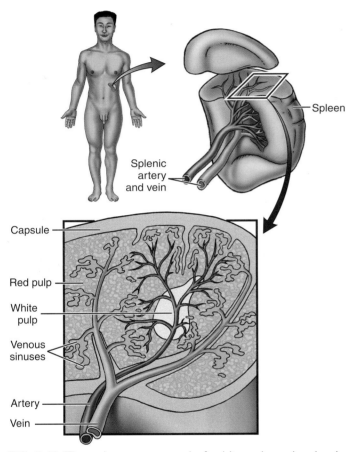

FIG. 2.10 The spleen, composed of white pulp and red pulp. (From Herlihy B: The human body in health and illness, ed 5, St Louis, 2014, Saunders.)

Esophageal Procedures

See Fig. 2.12. What parts of the anatomy are affected by these procedures?

- Esophagus
- Fundus of the stomach

Mapping

Here's the mapping for three procedures involving the esophagus:

SURGICAL MAPPING

Esophagectomy

Related Anatomy	Abnormal Anatomy	Pathology
Esophagus Fundus of the stomach	Narrowing of esophagus by tumor	Cancer

SURGICAL MAPPING

Esophagoduodenoscopy

Related Anatomy	Abnormal Anatomy	Pathology
Esophagus Stomach Duodenum	Stenosis esophagus Presences of polyps	Tumor Congenital Previous surgery

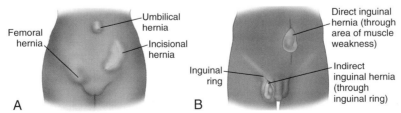

FIG. 2.11 Common types of abdominal hernias. **A,** Umbilical hernias result from a weakness in the abdominal wall around the umbilicus. An incisional hernia is herniation through inadequately healed surgery. In a femoral hernia, a loop of intestine descends through the femoral canal into the groin. **B,** Inguinal hernias are of two types. A *direct hernia* occurs through an area of weakness in the abdominal wall. In an *indirect hernia,* a loop of intestine descends through the inguinal canal, an opening in the abdominal wall for passage of the spermatic cord in males and a ligament of the uterus in females. (From Leonard PC: Building a medical vocabulary with Spanish translations, ed 9, St Louis, 2015, Saunders.)

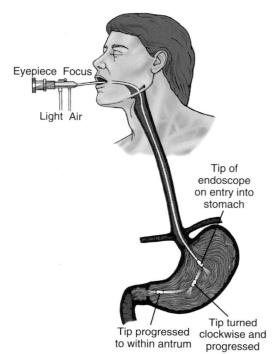

Eyepiece Focus

Light Air

Tip of
endoscope
on entry into
stomach

Tip turned
clockwise and
progressed

Tip progressed
to within antrum

FIG. 2.12 Example of flexible endoscopy. This endoscope is being used to examine the interior of the stomach through the esophagus. Depending on the structure to be examined, the physician chooses either a flexible or a rigid endoscope. Most of the interior stomach can be examined, including the antrum, located in the lower part of the stomach. (From Monahan FD, Neighbors M: Medical-surgical nursing: foundations for clinical practice, ed 2, Philadelphia, 1998, Saunders.)

SURGICAL MAPPING

Excision of esophageal diverticulum

Related Anatomy	Abnormal Anatomy	Pathology
Esophagus	Esophageal sac	Zenker's diverticulum (pharyngoesopha-geal diverticulum)

Stomach Procedures

What parts of the anatomy are affected by these surgeries?
- Stomach
- Duodenum
- Vagus nerve
- Jejunum (in some cases)
- Vagus nerve (cranial nerve X)

Mapping

Check out the maps of five common gastric procedures:

SURGICAL MAPPING

Vagotomy

Related Anatomy	Abnormal Anatomy	Pathology
Stomach Vagus nerve	Hypersecretion of hydrochloric acid in the stomach	Peptic ulcer

SURGICAL MAPPING

Billroth I

Related Anatomy	Abnormal Anatomy	Pathology
Stomach Duodenum	Damage to the stomach wall	Gastric carcinoma Benign tumor Chronic ulceration

SURGICAL MAPPING

Billroth II

Related Anatomy	Abnormal natomy	Pathology
Stomach Jejunum	Damage to the stomach wall	Benign tumor Chronic ulceration

SURGICAL MAPPING

Roux-en-Y gastric bypass

Related Anatomy	Abnormal natomy	Pathology
Stomach Duodenum Jejunum	No abnormality seen	Gastric ulcer Gastric carcinoma Morbid obesity

SURGICAL MAPPING

Gastrostomy

Related Anatomy	Abnormal Anatomy	Pathology
Stomach	No abnormality seen	Inability to feed normally because of debilitating condition

Small Intestine Procedures

What parts of the anatomy are affected by these procedures?
- Stomach
- Duodenum
- Jejunum
- Ileum
- Cecum

Mapping

Let's see how one procedure maps:

SURGICAL MAPPING

Meckel diverticulum removal

Related Anatomy	Abnormal Anatomy	Pathology
Distal ileum	Sac-like growth on the distal ileum	Congenital remnant of the umbilical duct

Large Intestine Procedures

See Fig. 2.13. What parts of the anatomy are affected by such procedures?
- Cecum
- Ascending colon

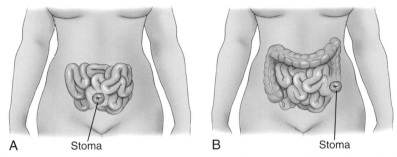

FIG. 2.13 Creation of an artificial opening in **A**, total colectomy and **B**, partial colectomy. (From LaFleur Brooks M, LaFleur Brooks D: Basic medical language, ed 5, St Louis, 2016, Elsevier.)

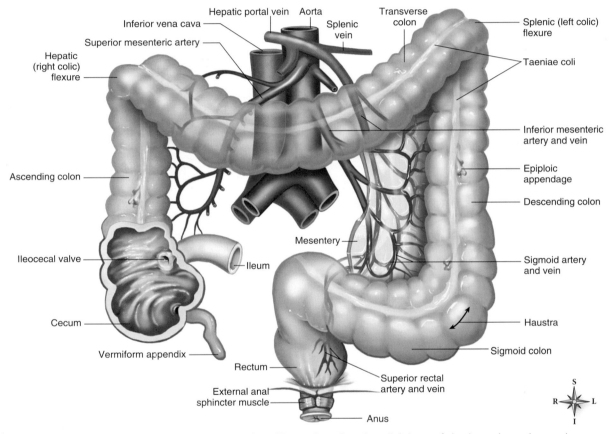

FIG. 2.14 Divisions of the large intestine. Illustration showing divisions of the large intestine and adjacent vascular structures. (From Patton KT, Thibodeau GA: Anatomy & physiology, ed 9, St Louis, 2016, Elsevier.)

- Transverse colon
- Descending colon
- Rectum
- Anus

Mapping

Let's collect the information you'll need to know about colectomy (Fig. 2.14), a surgery of the small intestine, and build a map:

SURGICAL MAPPING

Colectomy

Related Anatomy	Abnormal Anatomy	Pathology
Cecum	Inflammation of colon	Carcinoma
Ascending colon		Ulcerative colitis
Transverse colon		Perforated
Descending colon		diverticulum
Rectum		or recurrent
Anus		diverticulitis
Omentum		
Peritoneal covering of mesentery		
Appendix		

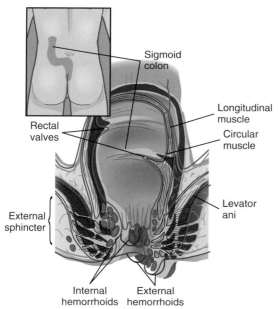

FIG. 2.15 Anatomical structures of the rectum and anus with external and internal hemorrhoids. (From Lewis SL, et al: Medical-surgical nursing: assessment and management of clinical problems, ed 9, St Louis, 2014, Mosby.)

Sigmoid and Rectal Procedures

What parts of the anatomy are affected by these procedures?

- Sigmoid
- Rectum
- Anus
- Large intestine
- Omentum
- Peritoneal covering of the mesentery
- Appendix

Mapping

Here's the basic information you'll need to know to assist at one procedure of the large intestine:

SURGICAL MAPPING

Sigmoidectomy/Low Anterior Resection

Related Anatomy	Abnormal Anatomy	Pathology
Sigmoid Rectum Anus	Inflammation of intestinal wall	Fistula Crohn disease

Anal Procedures

See Fig. 2.15. What parts of the anatomy may be affected by anal surgery?

- Sigmoid
- Rectum
- Anus
- Large intestine
- Omentum
- Peritoneal covering of the mesentery

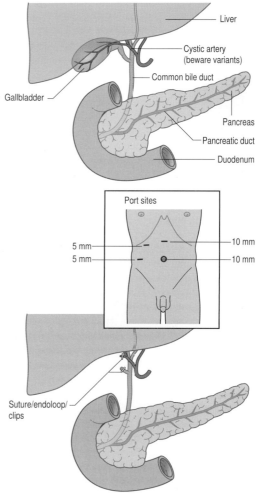

FIG. 2.16 Cholecystectomy. (From Franklin IJ, Dawson PM, Rodway AD: Pocket essentials of clinical surgery, ed 2, Edinburgh, 2012, Saunders.)

Mapping

Here's the map for one surgery of the anus.

SURGICAL MAPPING

Hemorrhoidectomy

Related Anatomy	Abnormal Anatomy	Pathology
Sigmoid Rectum Anus	Inflammation of blood vessels of anus Enlarged veins	Venous distention (varicose vein), often caused by obesity or pregnancy

Cholecystectomy

See Fig. 2.16. What parts of the anatomy are affected by cholecystectomy?

- Gallbladder
- Hepatic ducts
- Common bile ducts
- Cystic ducts

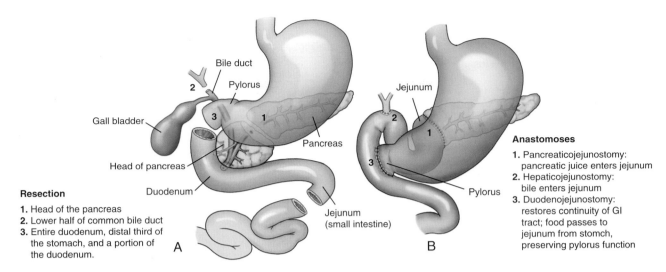

FIG. 2.17 Whipple procedure (pancreaticoduodenostomy).

Resection

1. Head of the pancreas
2. Lower half of common bile duct
3. Entire duodenum, distal third of the stomach, and a portion of the duodenum.

Anastomoses

1. Pancreaticojejunostomy: pancreatic juice enters jejunum
2. Hepaticojejunostomy: bile enters jejunum
3. Duodenojejunostomy: restores continuity of GI tract; food passes to jejunum from stomch, preserving pylorus function

SURGICAL MAPPING

Cholecystectomy (Removal of Gallbladder)

Related Anatomy	Abnormal Anatomy	Pathology
Gallbladder	Inflammation of gallbladder	Cholelithiasis
Hepatic ducts		
Common bile duct		
Cystic ducts		

Splenectomy

What parts of the anatomy are affected by splenectomy?

- Spleen
- Diaphragm
- Tail of pancreas
- Stomach
- Splenic artery
- Splenic vein

Mapping

The main procedure of the spleen is splenectomy: removal of the organ. Here's a map:

SURGICAL MAPPING

Splenectomy

Related Anatomy	Abnormal Anatomy	Pathology
Spleen	Splenomegaly	Abdominal trauma
Stomach		Blood disorders
Splenic artery		Cancer (e.g., leukemia,
Splenic vein		Hodgkin's lymphoma,
Diaphragm		spleen cancer, splenic
Tail of pancreas		laceration)
Splenorenal ligament		
Gastrosplenic ligament		

Whipple Procedure

See Fig. 2.17. What parts of the anatomy are affected by the Whipple procedure?

- Pancreas
- Duodenum
- Jejunum
- Ileum
- Stomach
- Large intestine
- Small intestine
- Hepatic bile ducts
- Common bile duct

Steps in Whipple Reconstruction

- The duodenum and a portion of the jejunum are removed, as is the proximal portion of the jejunum.
- The gastric omentum attachments are divided and the distal third of the stomach removed. The remaining stomach is attached to the jejunum in a side-to-side technique.
- The common bile duct (CBD) is divided just below the Y-junction of the cystic and hepatic ducts. An end-to-side technique is used to perform anastomosis of the CBD to the jejunum.
- The head of the pancreas is removed and anastomosis of the remaining portion of the pancreas to the jejunum is performed with the use of an end-to-end or side-to-side technique.

Mapping

Time to make a map!

SURGICAL MAPPING

Whipple Procedure (Pancreaticoduodenectomy)

Related Anatomy	Abnormal Anatomy	Pathology
Duodenum	Enlarged pancreas	Cancer of the head
Distal stomach		of the pancreas
Common bile duct		
Hepatic bile ducts		
Pancreatic duct		

Liver Procedures

See Fig. 2.18. What parts of the anatomy are affected by these procedures?

- Liver
- Inferior vena cava
- Gallbladder
- Common bile duct
- Hepatic bile ducts

SURGICAL MAPPING

Segmental resection

Related Anatomy	Abnormal Anatomy	Pathology
Liver	Enlarged liver	Benign tumor
Inferior vena cava		Malignant tumor
Gallbladder		Replacement of
Hepatic bile ducts		diseased liver
Common bile duct		
Pancreas		
Stomach		
Duodenum		
Jejunum		

SURGICAL MAPPING

Lobectomy

Related Anatomy	Abnormal Anatomy	Pathology
Liver	Enlarged liver●	
Inferior vena cava		
Gallbladder		
Hepatic bile ducts		
Common bile duct		
Pancreas		
Stomach		
Duodenum		
Jejunum		

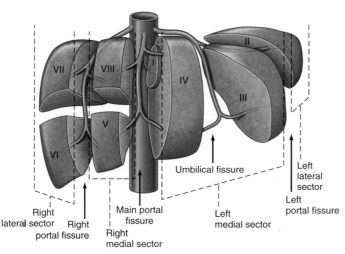

FIG. 2.18 The fissures and sectors of the liver. (Right lateral = right posterior; right medial = right anterior.) (From Standring S, ed: Gray's anatomy: the anatomical basis of clinical practice, ed 41, London, 2016, Elsevier.)

SURGICAL MAPPING

Liver transplant

Related Anatomy	Abnormal Anatomy	Pathology
Liver	Cirrhosis●	
Inferior vena cava		
Common bile duct		
Hepatic artery		
Portal vein		

The Breast

The breasts, secondary sex organs, are located high on the chest (Fig. 2.19). They are responsible for producing milk to nourish infants.

SURGICAL MAPPING

Mastectomy

Related Anatomy	Abnormal Anatomy	Pathology
Breast	Deformity	Cancer
Pectoralis major		
Pectoralis minor		
Axillary lymph nodes		

Breast Surgeries

What parts of the anatomy are affected by these procedures?

- Breast
- Deep fascia

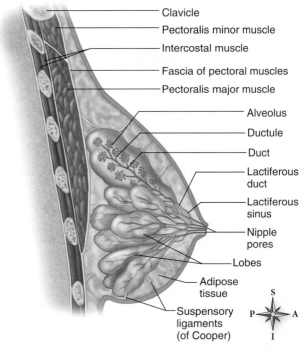

FIG. 2.19 Sagittal section of a lactating breast. Notice how the glandular structures are anchored to the overlying skin and to the pectoral muscles by the suspensory ligaments of Cooper. Each lobule of glandular tissue is drained by a lactiferous duct that eventually opens through the nipple. (From Patton KT, Thibodeau GA: Structure & function of the body, ed 15, St Louis, 2016, Elsevier.)

- Pectoralis major and minor
- Axillary lymph nodes (sentinel nodes)

Mapping

Let's assemble a map for one common treatment of breast cancer:

ENDOCRINE SYSTEM

Thyroid Gland

This organ secretes thyroid hormones, which regulate various body functions (Fig. 2.20):

- T3 (triiodothyronine)
- T4 (thyroxine)

What parts of the anatomy are affected by thyroid procedures?

- Thyroid
- Platysma
- Recurrent laryngeal nerve
- Parathyroid

Mapping

Let's map one common endocrine surgery:

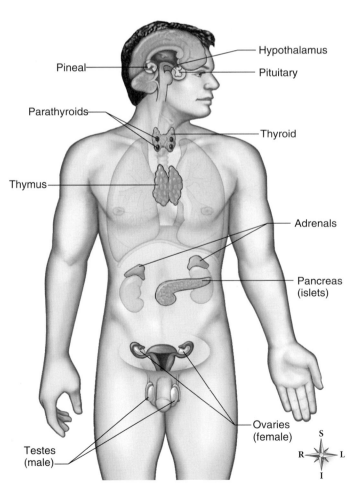

FIG. 2.20 Major endocrine glands. (From Patton KT, Thibodeau GA, Douglas MM: Essentials of Anatomy & Physiology, St Louis, 2012, Mosby.)

SURGICAL MAPPING

Thyroidectomy

Related Anatomy	Abnormal Anatomy	Pathology
Thyroid	Enlargement of thyroid gland	Goiter
Platysma		Airway obstruction
Recurrent laryngeal nerve		Graves disease
Parathyroid		Thyroid cancer

Parathyroid Gland

This organ regulates calcium through the secretion of parathyroid hormone.

What parts of the anatomy are affected by parathyroid surgeries?

- Thyroid
- Parathyroid gland
- Platysma
- Recurrent laryngeal nerve

Mapping

Let's pull together the information you'd need to know to assist in a parathyroid surgery:

SURGICAL MAPPING

Parathyroidectomy

Related Anatomy	Abnormal Anatomy	Pathology
Thyroid	Enlarged parathyroid gland	Parathyroid adenoma
Platysma		
Recurrent laryngeal nerve		
Parathyroid		

Adrenal Glands

What parts of the anatomy are affected by procedures of the adrenal glands?

- Adrenal glands
- Kidneys

Mapping

SURGICAL MAPPING

Adrenalectomy

Related Anatomy	Abnormal Anatomy	Pathology
Adrenal gland	Enlargement of adrenal gland	Pheochromocytoma
Kidney		Cushing syndrome
Suprarenal arteries		
Inferior vena cava		Adrenocortical carcinoma
Abdominal aorta		Hypersecretion of adrenocorticotropic hormone (ACTH)
Inferior phrenic arteries		

Ovaries

See Fig. 2.21. What parts of the anatomy are affected by surgery of the ovary?

- Ovary
- Fallopian tube
- Uterus

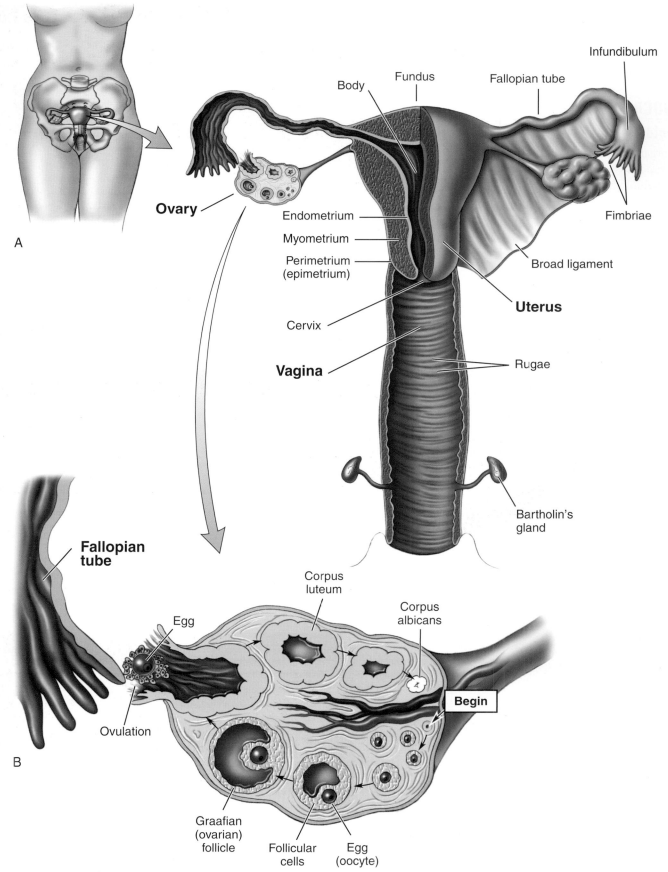

FIG. 2.21 A, Female reproductive organs. B, Maturation of the ovarian follicle, ovulation, and formation of the corpus luteum. (From Herlihy B: The human body in health and illness, ed 5, St Louis, 2014, Saunders.)

Mapping

Here's the map for oophorectomy (removal of an ovary).

SURGICAL MAPPING

SURGICAL MAPPING

Oophorectomy

Related Anatomy	Abnormal Anatomy	Pathology
Ovary	Enlarged ovary	Teratoma (dermoid cyst)
Fallopian tube		Polycystic ovary syndrome
Uterus		Benign or malignant tumor

Testicles

See Fig. 2.22. What parts of the anatomy are affected by surgeries of the testicles?

- Testes
- Scrotum
- Vas deferens

Mapping

Orchiectomy is the most commonly performed procedure of the testicle:

SURGICAL MAPPING

Orchiectomy

Related Anatomy	Abnormal Anatomy	Pathology
Scrotum	Enlarged testicle(s)	Torsion
Testes		Testicular carcinoma
Vas deferens		Trauma
Spermatic vessels		

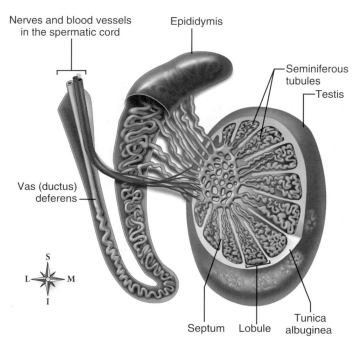

Nerves and blood vessels in the spermatic cord

Epididymis

Vas (ductus) deferens

Seminiferous tubules

Testis

Septum Lobule Tunica albuginea

FIG. 2.22 Tubules of the testis and epididymis. The ducts and tubules are exaggerated in size. (From Patton KT, Thibodeau GA: The Human Body in Health and Disease, ed 6, 2014, St Louis, Mosby.)

SURGICAL MAPPING

Hydrocelectomy

Related Anatomy	Abnormal Anatomy	Pathology
Scrotum	Fluid-filled scrotum	Trauma
Testicles		Infection
Vas deferens		Tumor
		Result of peritoneal dialysis

Pituitary Gland

This gland, found at the base of the brain, is divided into two sections (Fig. 2.23):

The **anterior pituitary** secretes many different hormones with a wide range of functions:

- Adrenocorticotrophic hormone (ACTH) causes the release of the hormones hydrocortisone (cortisol), aldosterone, and androgen. The most important of the three is cortisol. Hypersecretion of ACTH causes **Cushing syndrome**; hyposecretion of ACTH causes **Addison disease.**
- Thyroid-stimulating hormone (TSH) prompts the thyroid gland to produce **triiodothyronine** (T_3), which stimulates the metabolism of almost every tissue in the body.
- Luteinizing hormone (LH) is produced by gonadotropic cells in the anterior pituitary. An acute increase in LH triggers ovulation and development of the corpus luteum, essential for establishing and maintaining pregnancy. (The corpus luteum secretes progesterone, a steroid hormone responsible for the decidualization, or development, and maintenance of the endometrium. It also produces relaxin, a hormone responsible for softening of the pubic symphysis, which helps a woman give birth.)
- Follicle-stimulating hormone (FSH) stimulates the maturation of ovarian follicles.
- Prolactin (PRL) stimulates breast development and milk production.
- Growth hormone (GH), also known as somatotropin (or, in its human form, **human growth hormone [hGH or HGH]**), stimulates growth, cell reproduction, and cell regeneration in human beings and other animals.
- Melanocyte-stimulating hormone (MSH) prompts the production of the dark pigment melanin by cells known as skin cells called melanocytes. In human beings, melanocytes are responsible for moles, freckles, and suntan. (Cancerous lesions originating in the melanocytes are known as **melanomas.**)

The **posterior pituitary gland** also secretes hormones:

Oxytocin stimulates contractions during labor and then the production of milk and vasopressin (an antidiuretic hormone secreted by the pituitary gland) as posterior pituitary hormones are synthesized by the hypothalamus. These hormones are stored in neurosecretory vesicles (Herring bodies) before being secreted by the posterior pituitary into the bloodstream.

What parts of the anatomy are affected by procedures of the pituitary gland?

- Pituitary gland
- Hypothalamus
- Nasal cartilages

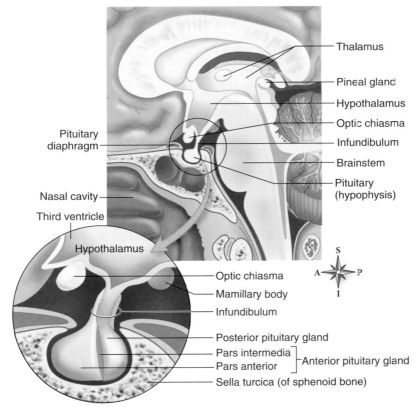

FIG. 2.23 Structure and location of the pituitary gland. (From Patton KT, Thibodeau GA, Douglas MM: Essentials of Anatomy & Physiology, St Louis, 2012, Mosby.)

Mapping

Here you can see how one pituitary surgery maps:

SURGICAL MAPPING

Transsphenoidal Hypophysectomy

Related Anatomy	Abnormal Anatomy	Pathology
Pituitary gland	Enlarged gland	Malignant
Nasal bones and cartilage		tumor
Sphenoid sinus		
Sella turcica		

INTEGUMENTARY SYSTEM

Skin

Knowledge of the integumentary system, particularly the skin, is important in the surgical setting, especially in regard to plastic and reconstructive surgery (Fig. 2.24).

The skin has several functions:

- It is the **first line of defense** against microorganisms.
- It is a **sensory** organ, registering touch, pressure, pain, and temperature.
- It **excretes** organic water and stores nutrients.

The skin comprises **two main layers**: the epidermis and the dermis. **Epidermis** is the outer layer of the skin, made up of cells called **keratinocytes**. New keratinocytes are being produced and pushed to the body's surface every day, just as dry, scaly dead cells are shed by the thousands each day.

The epidermis comprises five layers (*strata*):

- **Stratum basale**
  - *Basale* is Latin for "base"; this is the bottom layer of the epidermis.
  - This layer is also known as the *stratum germinativum*.
  - It is a reproductive layer, giving rise to keratinocytes.
  - Diffusion from capillaries in the dermis provides nourishment to this layer.
  - The stratum basale is also responsible for the production of melanin (pigment) for skin and hair.
- **Stratum spinosum**
  - *Spinosum* is Latin for "spiny"; the cells in this layer appear prickly or spiny because they have not yet differentiated into specialized cells.
  - This layer receives the daughter cells (keratinocytes).
- **Stratum granulosum**
  - Cells begin to flatten and take on a granular shape.
  - The process of keratinization begins here. (Keratin is a fibrous protein that makes up the hair, nails, and epidermis.)
- **Stratum lucidum**
  - This layer is only found on the palms and soles.
  - It's composed of dying or dead cells, flattened and densely packed.
  - It is appears translucent under a microscope, hence its name; *lucidum* is Latin for transparent.
- **Stratum corneum**
  - This is the most superficial layer.
  - It is composed of dead keratinocytes.

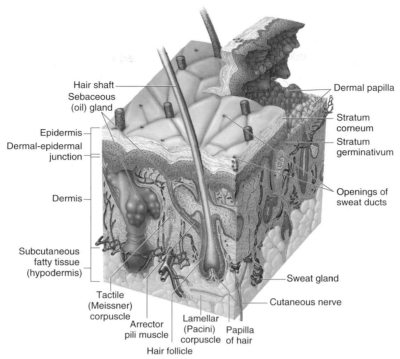

FIG. 2.24 Microscopic view of the skin. The epidermis, shown in longitudinal section, is raised at one corner to reveal the ridges in the dermis. (From Patton KT, Thibodeau GA: The Human Body in Health and Disease, ed 6, 2014, St Louis, Mosby.)

- It is thicker on such areas as the hands and feet.
- Cells in this layer are constantly shed, by the thousands, each day.

What parts of the anatomy are affected by procedures of the skin?
- Epidermis
- Dermis
- Subcutaneous fatty layer

Mapping

Here you can see how skin grafting maps:

SURGICAL MAPPING

Full- or Split-Thickness Skin Graft

Related Anatomy	Abnormal Anatomy	Pathology
Epidermis	Abnormal	Burns
Dermis	coloration	Basal cell carcinoma
Skin appendages		Trauma
		Infection (nonhealing ulcer, e.g., decubitus)

LYMPHATIC SYSTEM

See Fig. 2.25.

Tonsils and Adenoids

These lymphoid tissues serve as vital parts of the immune system.

What parts of the anatomy are affected by tonsil and adenoid procedures?
- Tonsils:
  - Palatine tonsils
  - Pharyngeal tonsils (adenoids)
- Mouth, including tongue, teeth, and uvula

Mapping

SURGICAL MAPPING

Tonsillectomy and adenoidectomy

Related Anatomy	Abnormal Anatomy	Pathology
Palatine tonsils (tonsil)	Hypertrophy of tonsil	Infection
Pharyngeal tonsils (adenoids)	and adenoids	Obstruction
		Recurrent tonsillitis
		Peritonsillar abscess

Thymus

See Fig. 2.26. What parts of the anatomy are affected by thymectomy (removal of the thymus)?
- Parietal pericardium
- Lungs
- Superior vena cava
- Brachiocephalic veins
- Common carotid artery

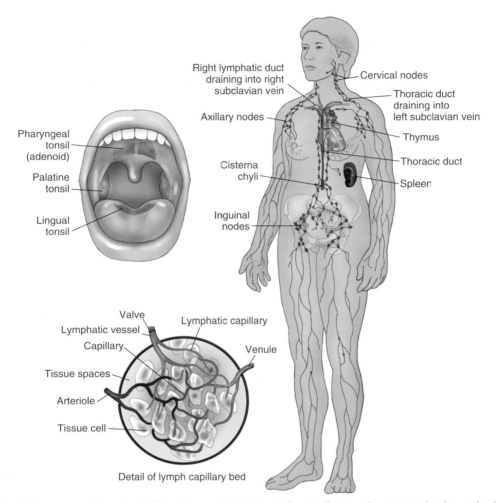

FIG. 2.25 Lymphatic system. The close relationship to the cardiovascular system is shown in the detailed drawing. Lymph capillaries merge to form lymphatic vessels that join other vessels to become trunks that drain large regions of the body. The right lymphatic duct receives fluid from the upper right quadrant of the body and empties into the right subclavian vein. The thoracic duct, which begins with the cisterna chyli, collects fluid from the rest of the body and empties it into the left subclavian vein. The lymph nodes are small, bean-shaped structures distributed along the vessels. Also shown are the lymphatic organs: tonsils, thymus, and spleen. (From Leonard PC: Building a medical vocabulary with Spanish translations, ed 9, St Louis, 2015, Saunders.)

Mapping

Here you can see how this procedure maps:

SURGICAL MAPPING		
Thymectomy		
Related Anatomy	**Abnormal Anatomy**	**Pathology**
Mediastinum	Enlargement of thymus	Thymoma
Parietal pericardium		
Lungs		
Common carotid artery		
Superior vena cava		

THE MUSCLES

Many procedures that we don't think of as involving muscles do, in fact, affect the muscular system to a great degree. We'll review three of them here.

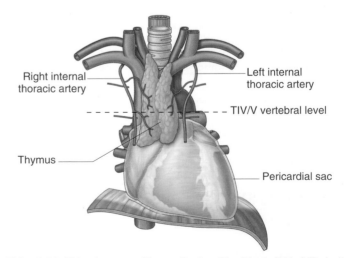

FIG. 2.26 The thymus. (From Drake RL, Vogl AW, Mitchell AWM: Gray's anatomy for students, ed 3, Philadelphia, 2015, Churchill Livingstone.)

Strabismus

See Fig. 2.27. What parts of the anatomy are affected by strabismus correction surgery?
- Extrinsic ocular muscles
- Bones of the orbit
- Conjunctiva
- Tenon's capsule

Mapping

Here are the basics of what you need to know about strabismus correction surgery.

SURGICAL MAPPING

Strabismus

Related Anatomy	Abnormal Anatomy	Pathology
Extrinsic ocular muscles	Misalignment of eyes	Esotropia ("crossed eyes")
Bones of the orbit		
Conjunctiva		Exotropia ("walleye")
Tenon's capsule		Amblyopia ("lazy eye")

Appendectomy

What parts of the anatomy are affected by this procedure?
- External oblique muscle
- Internal oblique muscle
- Transverse abdominis muscle

Mapping

Here you can see the anatomic basics of an appendectomy.

SURGICAL MAPPING

Appendectomy (Requiring Muscle-Splitting)

Related Anatomy	Abnormal Anatomy	Pathology
External oblique muscle	Inflamed appendix	Inflamed appendix
Internal oblique muscle	Ruptured appendix	Ruptured appendix
Transverse abdominis		
Peritoneum		

Nissen Fundoplication

See Fig. 2.28. What parts of the anatomy are affected by this procedure? (This is a gastric procedure, but think about the muscles that must be dissected to provide access to the stomach.)
- Right pillar of the crus
- Left pillar of the crus
- Posterior vagus nerve
- Fundus of the stomach

Mapping

Here we see the map for Nissen fundoplication.

SURGICAL MAPPING

Nissen Fundoplication

Related Anatomy	Abnormal Anatomy	Pathology
Right and left pillars of the crus	Protrusion of fundus of stomach into thoracic cavity	Hiatal hernia
Posterior vagus nerve		Gastroesophageal reflux disease (GERD_
Fundus of the stomach		

NEUROLOGICAL SYSTEM

Cranial Nerves

One of the most important parts of the nervous system that you'll need to be able to recall on your certification exam is cranial nerve system, comprising these 12 nerves (Fig. 2.29):
- **Cranial nerve I (olfactory nerve)** is responsible for the sense of smell.
- **Cranial nerve II (optic nerve)** conveys impulses for sight.
- **Cranial nerve III (oculomotor nerve)** controls the muscle that moves the eye and the iris.
- **Cranial nerve IV (trochlear nerve)** controls the oblique muscle of the eye.
- **Cranial nerve V (trigeminal nerve)** controls sensation in the face (forehead, mouth, nose, and top of the head).
- **Cranial nerve VI (abducens nerve)** controls lateral movement of the eye.

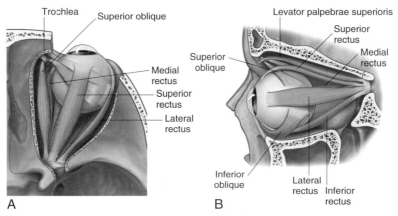

FIG. 2.27 Muscles of the eyeball. **A,** Superior view. **B,** Lateral view. (From Drake RL, Vogl AW, Mitchell AWM: Gray's anatomy for students, ed 3, Philadelphia, 2015, Churchill Livingstone.)

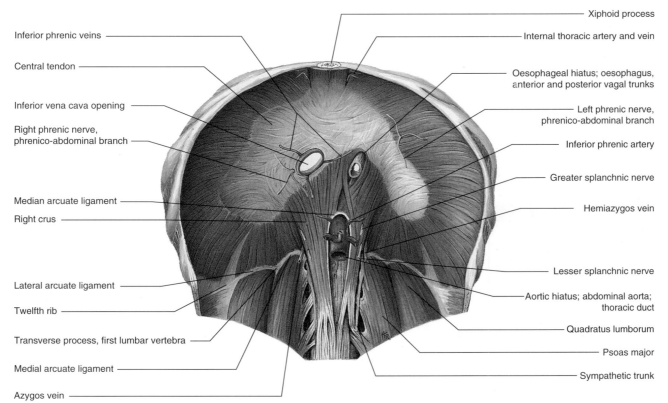

FIG. 2.28 Abdominal aspect of the diaphragm. Note the apertures for the esophagus and inferior vena cava and the aortic hiatus. The medial part of the right crus frequently consists of three components and extends further distally than the left crus. (Printed with permission from Waschke J, Paulsen F [eds], Sobotta Atlas of Human Anatomy, 15th ed, Elsevier, Urban & Fischer. Copyright 2013.)

- **Cranial nerve VII (facial nerve)** controls the muscles of the face and scalp, as well as tearing and salivation.
- **Cranial nerve VIII (vestibulocochlear [acoustic] nerve)** controls hearing and equilibrium.
- **Cranial nerve IX (glossopharyngeal nerve)** controls the sense of taste, pharyngeal movement, and parotid salivation.
- **Cranial nerve X (vagus nerve)** innervates the pharyngeal and laryngeal muscles, heart, pancreas, lungs, and digestive system.
- **Cranial nerve XI (accessory nerve)** comprises two parts:
  - The *cranial portion* joins with the vagus nerve to help control pharyngeal and laryngeal muscles.
  - The *spinal portion* controls the trapezius and sternocleidomastoid muscles.
- **Cranial nerve XII (hypoglossal nerve)** innervates the muscle of the tongue.

Layers of the Head

The process of cutting into the brain involves these layers, starting with the skin and working inward:

- Skin
- Fat
- Periosteum
- Bone
- Dura mater
- Arachnoid mater
- Pia mater

Craniotomy

What parts of the anatomy are affected by this procedure?
- Skin
- Fat
- Periosteum
- Bone
- Dura mater
- Arachnoid mater
- Pia mater
- Subdural space
- Cerebrospinal fluid

Mapping

Here's the map for craniotomy:

SURGICAL MAPPING		
Craniotomy		
Related Anatomy	**Abnormal Anatomy**	**Pathology**
Skin	Destruction of brain tissue	Malignant tumor
Fat	Compression of nerve	(e.g., glioma)
Periosteum	tissue	Benign tumors
Bone		(e.g., hemangioma)
Dura mater Arachnoid mater Pia mater		Brain injury
Subdural space		Brain abscess
Cerebrospinal fluid		

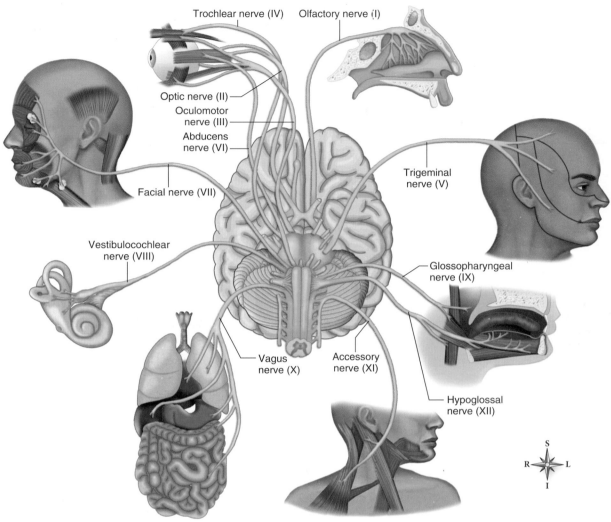

FIG. 2.29 Cranial nerves. View of the undersurface of the brain shows attachments of the cranial nerves. (From Patton KT, Thibodeau GA: The Human Body in Health and Disease, ed 6, 2014, St Louis, Mosby.)

Carpal Tunnel Release

What parts of the anatomy are affected by this procedure?
- Median nerve
- Transverse carpal ligament
- Skin
- Fat
- Erector spinae muscle
- Lamina

Mapping

Let's map our procedure:

SURGICAL MAPPING

Carpal tunnel release

Related Anatomy	Abnormal Anatomy	Pathology
Skin	Compression of median	Repetitive
Transverse carpal ligament	nerve by transverse	strain
Median nerve	carpal ligament	

Laminectomy

See Fig. 2.30. What parts of the anatomy are affected by this procedure? (Focus on the layers that are involved.)

Mapping

Laminectomy is one common spinal procedure:

SURGICAL MAPPING

Laminectomy

Related Anatomy	Abnormal Anatomy	Pathology
Skin	Compression	Lumbar spondylosis
Fat	of spinal nerve	Lumbar stenosis
Erector spinae		Lumbar
Lamina		spondylolisthesis
		Diskectomy

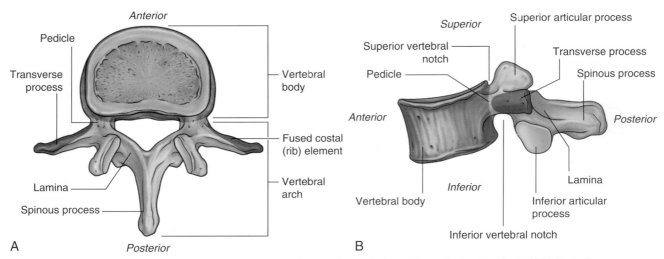

FIG. 2.30 A typical vertebra. **A,** Superior view. **B,** Lateral view. (From Drake RL, Vogl AW, Mitchell AWM: Gray's anatomy for students, ed 3, Philadelphia, 2015, Churchill Livingstone.)

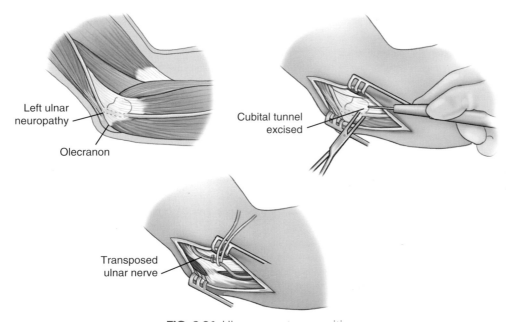

FIG. 2.31 Ulnar nerve transposition.

Ulnar Nerve Transposition

What parts of the anatomy are affected by this procedure? (Think about the layers that the surgeon must go through and the position of the nerve before and after the surgery [Fig. 2.31].)

- Ulnar nerve
- Ligament of Osborne
- Guyon canal

Mapping

This is how ulnar nerve transposition maps:

SURGICAL MAPPING

Ulnar nerve transposition

Related Anatomy	Abnormal Anatomy	Pathology
Ulnar nerve	Compression or entrap-	Repetitive strain
Ligament of Osborne	ment of ulnar nerve	injury
Guyon canal		Accidental bumping of epicondyle of elbow

PERIPHERAL VASCULAR SYSTEM

As you know, the two main divisions of blood vessels are arteries and veins (Fig. 2.32). Before moving on to map a couple of surgeries involving the blood vessels, let's review their structure, function, and other characteristics (Table 2.1).

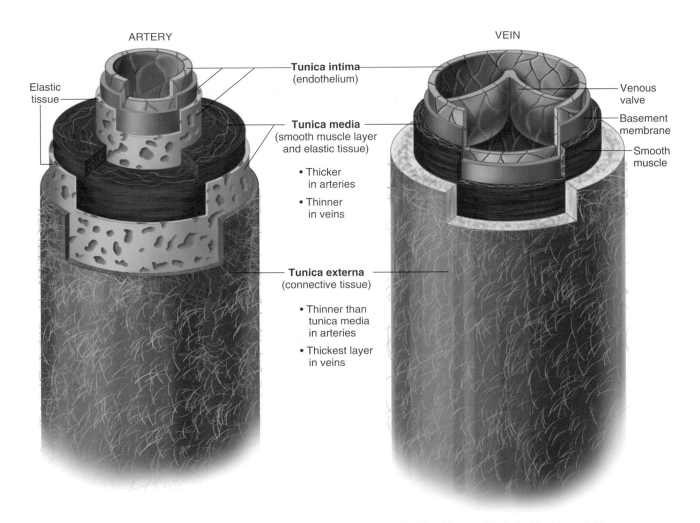

ARTERY

VEIN

Elastic
tissue

Tunica intima
(endothelium)

Venous
valve

Basement
membrane

Smooth
muscle

Tunica media
(smooth muscle layer
and elastic tissue)

• Thicker
  in arteries

• Thinner
  in veins

Tunica externa
(connective tissue)

• Thinner than
  tunica media
  in arteries

• Thickest layer
  in veins

FIG. 2.32 Artery and vein. (From Patton KT, Thibodeau GA: The Human Body in Health and Disease, ed 6, 2014, St Louis, Mosby.)

TABLE 2.1	**Differences Between Arteries and Veins**	
Characteristics	**Arteries**	**Veins**
Layers	Tunica adventitia (externa)	Tunica adventitia (inner)
	Tunica media (middle; thick, elastic)	Tunica media (middle; thin, nonelastic)
	Tunica intima (inner)	Tunica intima (inner)
Function	Carries oxygen from the heart to various parts of the body (with the exception of the pulmonary artery, which carries deoxygenated blood from heart to lungs)	Carries deoxygenated blood from various parts of body to heart (with the exception of the pulmonary vein, which carries oxygenated blood from lungs to heart)
Valves	Absent	Present (to stop backflow of blood)
Blood flow pressure	High	Low

Carotid Endarterectomy

See Fig. 2.33. What parts of the anatomy are affected by this procedure? (Focus on the artery involved.)

• Common carotid artery
• Internal carotid artery

Mapping

Here's how the surgery maps:

SURGICAL MAPPING

Carotid endarterectomy

Related Anatomy	**Abnormal Anatomy**	**Pathology**
Common carotid artery	Carotid stenosis	Accumulation
Internal carotid artery		of plaque
		Atherosclerosis

Arteriovenous Fistula and Shunt

One of the most commonly performed dialysis shunt procedures is the Cimino fistula (Fig. 2.34A).

What parts of the anatomy are affected by this procedure? (Focus on the artery and vein involved.)

- Radial artery
- Cephalic vein

Mapping

Now let's break the shunt procedure into its components.

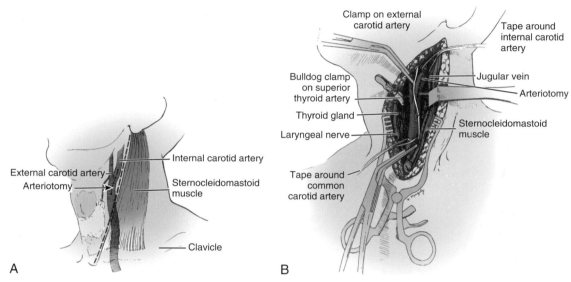

FIG. 2.33 Left carotid endarterectomy. **A,** Incision and anatomy. **B,** Exposure of carotid bifurcation. (From Hershey FB, Calman CH: *Atlas of vascular surgery,* ed 3, St Louis, 1973, Mosby.)

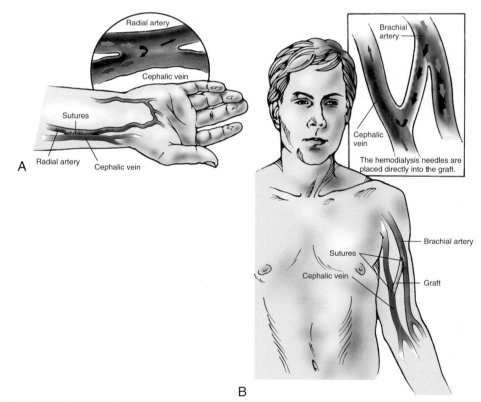

FIG. 2.34 **A,** A surgically created venous fistula. The increased pressure from the artery forces blood into the vein. This process causes the vein to dilate enough for fistula needles to be placed for hemodialysis. When the vein dilates in this matter, the fistula is said to be "developed." **B,** A surgically placed straight vascular graft in the upper arm. The graft creates a shunt between arterial and venous blood. (From Ignatavicius DD, Workman ML: Medical-surgical nursing: critical thinking for collaborative care, ed 6, St. Louis, 2010, Saunders.)

Arteriovenous fistula and shunt (Cimino fistula)

Related Anatomy	Abnormal Anatomy	Pathology
Radial artery Cephalic vein	None	Kidney failure necessitating long-term dialysis

Abdominal Aortic Aneurysm Repair

What parts of the anatomy are affected by this procedure? (Focus on the arteries involved.)

- Abdominal aorta
- Common iliac artery

Mapping

Let's see how this surgery maps:

SURGICAL MAPPING

Abdominal aortic aneurysm repair

Related Anatomy	Abnormal Anatomy	Pathology
Abdominal aorta Common iliac artery	Weakening of arterial wall	Atherosclerosis Aneurysm

REPRODUCTIVE SYSTEM

Female Reproductive System

See Figs. 2.35 and 2.36. The female reproductive tract consists of the:

- Ovaries (which are also considered part of the endocrine system because they secrete hormones)
- Fallopian (uterine) tubes
- Uterus
- Cervix
- Vagina

- Vulva
- Labia majora
- Labia minora
- Clitoris
- Vestibule
- Hymen
- Bartholin glands

Hysterectomy

What parts of the anatomy are affected by this procedure? (Focus on the ligaments and other structures involved.)

- Round ligament
- Uterine ligament
- Broad ligaments
- Cardinal ligament
- Uterus
- Cervix
- Iliac artery

Mapping

Here are the anatomic basics of what you need to know about hysterectomy:

SURGICAL MAPPING

Hysterectomy

Related Anatomy	Abnormal Anatomy	Pathology
Round ligament Uterine ligament Broad ligaments Cardinal ligament Uterus Cervix Iliac artery	Abnormal bleeding Presence of fibroid	Postmenopausal bleeding Endometriosis Cancer

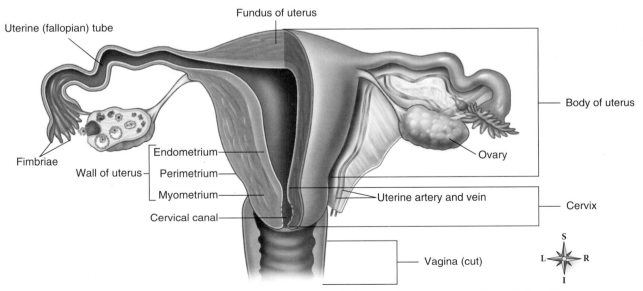

FIG. 2.35 The uterus. Sectioned view shows muscle layers of the uterus and its relationship to the ovaries and vagina. (From Patton KT, Thibodeau GA: Structure & function of the body, ed 15, St Louis, 2016, Elsevier.)

Male Reproductive System

See Fig. 2.37. The organs and structures required for reproduction in the male are the:

- Testicles
- Scrotum
- Epididymis
- Vas deferens
- Seminal vesicles
- Prostate gland
- Bulbourethral glands
- Penis

Now it's your turn! Use the template to map this common procedure of the male reproductive tract:

- Vasectomy

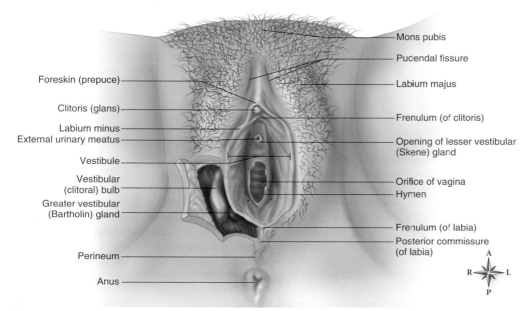

FIG. 2.36 External genitals of the female. (From Patton KT, Thibodeau GA: Structure & function of the body, ed 15, St Louis, 2016, Elsevier.)

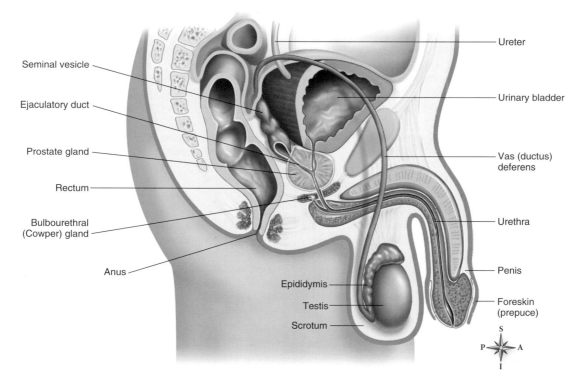

FIG. 2.37 Organization of the male reproductive organs. (From Patton KT, Thibodeau GA: Structure & function of the body, ed 15, St Louis, 2016, Elsevier.)

CONCLUSION

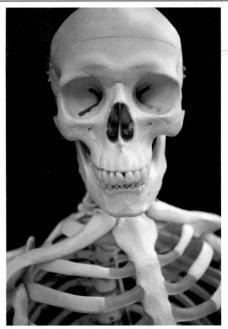

(Copyright © PeskyMonkey/iStock/Getty Images.)

You've completed this review of anatomy and how it relates to common surgical procedures. If you feel ready, complete the chapter review questions and check your answers in the Answer Key at the back of the book. If you feel that you need more work, make your way through the chapter again. Visit the Evolve Resources site for additional practice.

REVIEW QUESTIONS

1. The _____ is the lining of the inner wall of the heart's chambers.
   a. Pericardium
   b. Endocardium
   c. Epicardium
   d. Myocardium

2. The heart's natural pacemaker is situated atop the:
   a. Right ventricle
   b. Right atrium
   c. Left atrium
   d. Left ventricle

3. _____ is the result of electrical stimulation of the heart.
   a. Cardiac relaxation
   b. Partial filling with deoygenated blood
   c. Cardiac polarity
   d. Cardiac contraction

4. Identify the manner in which electricity passes through the atria in a wavelike motion:
   a. Ventricular contraction stimulates the AV (atrioventricular) node, and then the impulse passes on to the ventricles by traveling through the bundle of His, bundle branches, and Purkinje fibers lying in the muscle of the ventricles.
   b. Relaxation of the right atrium stimulates the AV node; then the impulse is passed on to the ventricles, traveling through the bundle of His and stopping.
   c. Atrial contraction of the right atrium stimulates the AV node then passes on to the ventricles, traveling through the bundle of His, bundle branches, and Purkinje fibers lying in the muscle of the ventricles.
   d. The AV node, which is the natural pacemaker of the heart, passes the impulse on to the ventricles; it travels through the bundle of His, bundle branches, and Purkinje fibers lying in the muscle of the ventricles.

5. The _____ is located between the right atrium and the right ventricle.
   a. Bicuspid
   b. Tricuspid valve
   c. Mitral valve
   d. Aortic valve

6. The _____ is located between the left ventricle and the aorta.
   a. Aortic valve
   b. Semilunar valve
   c. Mitral valve
   d. Pulmonary valve

7. The _____ is located between the left atrium and the left ventricle.
   a. Pulmonary valve
   b. Tricuspid valve
   c. Aortic valve
   d. Mitral valve

8. Leakage of a valve is known as:
   a. Atresia
   b. Stenosis
   c. Regurgitation
   d. Prolapse

9. The condition in which a valve opening hasn't developed at all, preventing blood from passing from an atrium to a ventricle or from a ventricle to the pulmonary artery or aorta, is called:
   a. Atresia
   b. Stenosis
   c. Regurgitation
   d. Arteriosclerosis

10. This thick layer of the digestive tract contains nerve plexus, blood vessels, and glands.
    a. Mucosa
    b. Submucosa
    c. Serosa
    d. Muscularis

11. The mesentery that connects the greater curvature of the stomach to the transverse colon and posterior body wall is called the:
    a. Parietal peritoneum
    b. Lesser omentum
    c. Serous membrane
    d. Greater omentum

12. All of following organs are considered retroperitoneal organs **except** the:
    a. Duodenum
    b. Rectum
    c. Stomach
    d. Urinary bladder

13. This thin fold of tissue is part of the tongue.
    a. Gums
    b. Teeth
    c. Lips
    d. Frenulum

14. Adults normally have _____ permanent teeth; children have _____ deciduous teeth.
    a. 31; 32
    b. 32; 20
    c. 32; 32
    d. 32; 36

15. The center of each tooth, filled with blood vessels, nerves, and connective tissue, is called:
    a. Pulp
    b. Gums
    c. Cementum
    d. Dentin

16. The living cellular and calcified dental tissue that surrounds the pulp cavity is known as:
    a. Pulp
    b. Dentin
    c. Enamel
    d. Cementum

17. Amylase is found in the:
    a. Esophagus and stomach
    b. Duodenum and pylorus
    c. Pancreas and salivary gland
    d. Thyroid and parathyroid glands

18. Which of the following is **not** one of the three pairs of extrinsic salivary glands?
    a. Palatine
    b. Parotid
    c. Submandibular
    d. Sublingual

19. Bile is produced by the _____ and secreted into the bile canaliculi.
    a. Liver lobules
    b. Gallbladder
    c. Common bile duct
    d. Hepatocytes

20. The main part of the stomach is called the:
    a. Body
    b. Cardiac stomach
    c. Esophageal sphincter muscle
    d. Fundus

21. The main job of the large intestine is:
    a. To digest food
    b. To control gas-producing microorganisms
    c. To remove toxins
    d. To eliminate feces

22. The salivary enzyme amylase begins the digestion of:
    a. Fats
    b. Carbohydrates
    c. Amino acids
    d. Proteins

23. The least bacteria are found in the:
    a. Large intestine
    b. Small intestine
    c. Stomach
    d. Appendix

24. Name the gastrointestinal layers, from outside to inside:
    a. Muscular layer, submucosa, mucosa, serosa
    b. Submucosa, mucosa, serosa, muscular layer
    c. Serosa, submucosa, mucosa, muscular layer
    d. Serosa, muscular layer, submucosa, mucosa

25. The appendix is located at the:
    a. Descending colon
    b. Ileum
    c. Cecum
    d. Ascending colon

26. *Escherichia coli* produces vitamin:
    a. B12
    b. K
    c. C
    d. D

27. The gallbladder is located in the angle between the linea semilunaris and the:
    a. Right lower quadrant
    b. Right costal margin
    c. Right side of the stomach
    d. Right side of the duodenum

28. This organ is an exocrine and endocrine gland and has a head, neck, body, and tail:
    a. Spleen
    b. Gallbladder
    c. Stomach
    d. Pancreas

29. A 1-month-old boy is brought to the emergency department with projectile vomiting and constant crying. Which part of the infant's stomach is involved?
    a. Rugae
    b. Fundus
    c. Pylorus
    d. Body

30. During splenectomy, the tail of the pancreas, which is closely associated with the spleen, is located and preserved. What is the name of the ligament associated with this structure?

a. Gastrosplenic ligament
b. Splenorenal ligament
c. Phrenicocolic ligament
d. Gastrocolic ligament

31. The esophagus lies _____ to the trachea.
    a. Anterior
    b. Lateral
    c. Posterior
    d. Medial

32. The opening in the diaphragm that allows the esophagus to pass through and connect to the stomach is known as the _____ hiatus.
    a. Esophageal
    b. Mediastinal
    c. Thoracic
    d. Diaphragmatic

33. All of the following organs produce hormones in addition to their major functions **except** the:
    a. Pancreas
    b. Pituitary
    c. Kidneys
    d. Thymus

34. The largest organ in the body is the:
    a. Liver
    b. Skin
    c. Lung
    d. Brain

35. Melanin is responsible for coloring both:
    a. Skin and nails
    b. Skin and irises
    c. Skin and hair
    d. Skin and pupils

36. A 3-year-old child is brought to the emergency department with third-degree burns. Which part of the skin is destroyed?
    a. Only the epidermis
    b. Epidermis and dermis
    c. Epidermis and some of the dermis
    d. Only the dermis

37. All of these arteries carry oxygen-rich blood **except** the:
    a. Femoral artery
    b. Aorta
    c. Pulmonary artery
    d. Mesenteric artery

38. The layers of a blood vessel, from outside to innermost, are:
    a. Adventitia, intima, media
    b. Intima, media, adventitia
    c. Media, adventitia, intima
    d. Adventitia, media, intima

39. Systolic pressure is recorded when the:
    a. Ventricle relaxes
    b. Ventricle contracts
    c. Atrium relaxes
    d. Atrium contracts

40. The innermost layer of the uterus is the:
    a. Myometrium
    b. Perimetrium
    c. Endometrium
    d. Epimetrium

41. What is the name of the erectile tissue in the female that corresponds to the corpus spongiosum in the male?
    a. Bulb of the vestibule
    b. Labia majora
    c. Prepuce
    d. Clitoris

42. The primary sex organ in males is the:
    a. Scrotum
    b. Penis
    c. Prepuce
    d. Testes

43. A patient is scheduled for a vasectomy. Which of these structures will be removed during this procedure?
    a. Vas deferens
    b. Ejaculatory duct
    c. Seminal vesicles
    d. Urethra

44. *Ectopic pregnancy* is the term used to describe a pregnancy that does not occur within the uterus. In which part of the reproductive system is ectopic pregnancy commonly seen?
    a. Fimbriae
    b. Fallopian tube
    c. Ovarian tube
    d. Vaginal vault

45. The _____ is found between the uterus and the vagina.
    a. Hymen
    b. Vulva
    c. Urethra
    d. Cervix

46. The hormone that stimulates uterine contractions is:
    a. Oxytocin
    b. Progesterone
    c. Adrenaline
    d. Estrogen

47. The outermost layer of the meninges is the:
    a. Meningioma
    b. Pia mater
    c. Dura mater
    d. Arachnoid mater

48. The respiratory center is located in the:
    a. Medulla oblongata and midbrain
    b. Medulla oblongata and pons
    c. Pons only
    d. Medulla oblongata only

49. The outermost layer of each kidney is called the:
    a. Renal pelvis
    b. Renal pyramid
    c. Renal medulla
    d. Renal cortex

50. The renal artery, renal vein, and ureter enter the kidney through the:
    a. Hilum
    b. Renal sinus
    c. Renal cortex
    d. Renal pelvis

Surgical Environment

As you know, modern surgery involves an almost dizzying array of equipment and rules for keeping it all clean to prevent infection. In this chapter, we'll review all facets of the surgical environment: setting, electronic and non-electronic equipment, and cleansing techniques.

OPERATING ROOM ENVIRONMENT

The surgical department must be set up in a way that fosters efficiency.

- The "racetrack" layout favored by many facilities (Fig. 3.1A) consists of a central area surrounded by several operating rooms. It permits the flow of patient traffic from the preoperative holding area to an operating room and, finally, to in the post-anesthesia care unit (PACU).
- The "hotel" layout (Fig. 3.1B) comprises a central hallway that has, on each side, one or more operating rooms plus the scrub, substerile, and supply rooms needed to run them.
- The central corridor layout (Fig. 3.1C) consists of a large central corridor with operating rooms and their sterile and scrub areas on each side. Rooms for supplies and equipment are placed in the middle of the large corridor, giving the corridor a racetrack, appearance.

Areas of the Surgical Department

The surgical department comprises three main areas, delineated by degree of cleanliness and type of clothing required:

- ***Restricted area.*** Operating rooms and sterile core areas (e.g., sterile stocking) require personnel to wear a scrub suit, hat, mask, and booties.
- ***Semi-restricted area.*** Usually a red line separates the semi-restricted area, which includes the nursing desk and hallway into the OR, from the unrestricted area. Surgical scrubs, hat, and booties are required.
- ***Unrestricted area:*** In the perioperative holding area (waiting room), street clothes may be worn

Operating Room

The operating room, of course, is the room in which surgical interventions are performed (Fig. 3.2).

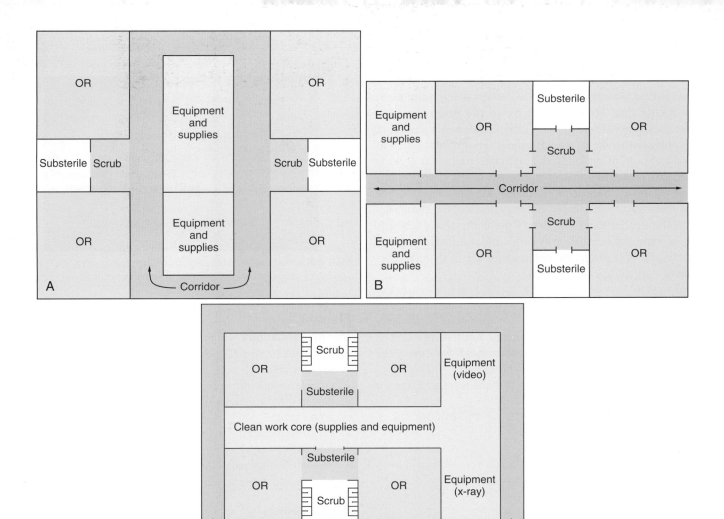

FIG. 3.1 Surgical department layouts. A, Central corridor, racetrack style. B, Central corridor, hotel style. C, Central core, peripheral corridor style. (From Phillips N: Berry & Kohn's operating room technique, ed 13, St Louis, 2017, Elsevier.)

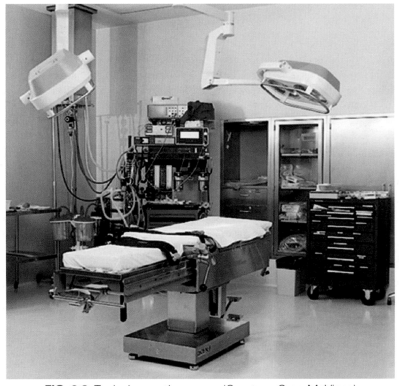

FIG. 3.2 Typical operating room. (Courtesy Greg McVicar.)

Specifications

- Humidity is maintained at 20% to 60%. (A humidity reading higher than 60% is conducive to the development of static electricity; a reading lower than 20% means that spark transmission is likely.) These standards were established as an aid to preventing fire in the operating room. Controlling humidity also limits microbial growth in the OR, prevents electrostatic discharge (ESD), and ensures the comfort of the OR team. Over time, these concerns have eased somewhat with the development and use of nonflammable anesthetic gases, improved ventilation systems, and the development of flame- and ESD-retardant materials for use in the manufacture of sterile drapes and gowns.
- Temperature is maintained at 68° to 73° F in most cases but is kept higher for pediatric, trauma, and immunosuppressed patients.
- Laminar air flow with unidirectional positive pressure is used in some hospitals to prevent microbes from leaving the OR or entering the surgical suite.
- There's one suction outlet for the surgical team and one for anesthesia.
- Gas outlets are color-coded for safety and ease of use:
  - *Blue:* nitrous oxide
  - *Black:* nitrogen
  - *Green:* oxygen
  - *Gray:* carbon dioxide
  - *Yellow:* compressed air
- Furniture includes:
  - Operating table
  - Back table
  - Mayo stand
  - Ring stand
  - Kick buckets
  - OR lights

Decontamination Room

Gross decontamination (removal of visible debris) is performed in this utility area, which is located in the semi-restricted area. The decontamination room holds specimens awaiting transport to the laboratory and is where instrumentation is washed before immediate-use steam sterilization for return to the sterile field.

SURGICAL INSTRUMENTATION

Countless instruments are used in modern surgery (Fig. 3.3). We'll touch on a few that you'll be expected to know on your certification exam (Table 3.1).

ELECTROSURGICAL EQUIPMENT

Not all surgery is accomplished with the use of scalpels, forceps, clamps, and needles alone. These days, much of it requires electronic equipment whose use you must be familiar with.

Before we move on to the various types of electronic surgical equipment and their purposes, let's quickly review some pertinent electrical terms and their definitions (Table 3.2).

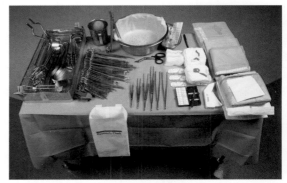

FIG. 3.3 Basic back table setup. (From Tighe SM: Instrumentation for the operating room: a photographic manual, ed 9, St Louis, 2016, Mosby.)

Electrocautery

Monopolar Cautery

Monopoloar cautery (Fig. 3.4) is the most commonly used type of electrocautery.

- Offers coagulation, cut, and blend modes
- Powered by a generator (a.k.a. Bovie machine, monopolar power unit)
- Performed with the use of a sterile active electrode (cautery pencil)
- Nonsterile dispersive electrode attached to patient to disperse current and prevent injury

Bipolar Cautery

Another type of electrocautery is bipolar cautery (Fig. 3.5).

- Powered by a generator or other power
- Performed with the use of an active electrode and (sterile) bipolar forceps
- Current passes through tissue grasped within the forceps, then returns to the generator through the tip of the forceps (Fig. 3.4)

Other Electrocautery Devices

- *Argon beam.* Argon, an inert gas, is incapable of combustion but permits passage of electrical current. A special argon beam grounding pad is required for the patient.
- *Harmonic scalpel.* This device uses ultrasonic energy to cut and coagulate tissue. No grounding pad is needed.
- *CUSA (Cavitron Ultrasonic Surgical Aspirator).* This patented device uses ultrasonic energy to emulsify and aspirate tissue. No grounding pad is needed.

Electrocautery Safety Tips

- Apply the grounding pad to a large fleshy area that is clean and dry (e.g., the thigh).
- Never place a grounding pad on a bony area or prominence or over a metal prosthesis.
- Never let skin prep solutions or other liquids pool around a grounding pad.
- Ensure that the grounding pad is placed in full contact with skin—no wrinkling or tunneling.
- Place the grounding pad as close to the surgical site as possible.
- Remove all jewelry and other metal objects from the patient before surgery.

Continued on following page 52

TABLE 3.1 Basic Surgical Instrumentation

Instrument	Use
Knife Handles	
#3 (fits #10, #11, #12, and #15 blades)	Cutting and dissecting
#4 (fits #21, #21, and #23 blades)	Cutting and dissecting
#7 (fits #10, #11, #12, and #15 blades)	Cutting and dissecting
Scissors	
Mayo, straight	Suture scissors
Mayo, curved	Dissecting tough tissue
Metzenbaum	Delicate dissection
Potts-Smith	Cardiovascular work
Iris	Gentle dissection for neurological, ophthalmologic, and plastic surgery
Stevens tenotomy	Gentle dissection in neurological, ophthalmologic, and plastic surgery
Bone-shaping Tools	
Chisels	Shaping bone
Osteotomes	Cutting bone
Gouges	Channeling, cutting, or scooping bone
Rasps	Filing and shaping bone
Forceps	
Toothed tissue	Grasping and holding tough tissue
Adson tissue	Grasping and holding delicate tissue
Bishop Harmon tissue	Grasping and holding delicate tissue
Russian tissue	Grasping and holding tough tissue
Allis	Toothed for grasping
Kocher	Toothed for grasping
Babcock	Smooth for grasping delicate tissue
Tenaculum Forceps	
Lahey	Thyroid-grasping clamp

Schroeder	Single-toothed tenaculum for grasping and holding tissue

Continued

TABLE 3.1   Basic Surgical Instrumentation—cont'd

Instrument	Use
Jacob	Double-toothed for grasping and holding tissue

Bone Clamps

Lane	Grasping and holding bone

Lowman	Grasping and holding bone

Hemostatic Forceps

Mosquito	Clamping and occluding small vessels
Crile	Grasping larger vessels or tissue
Mixter	Right-angle forceps for grasping or clamping
Tonsil (Adson or Schnidt)	Locking forceps for controlling bleeding

Intestinal Clamps

Allen	Grasping or occluding tissue

TABLE 3.1 Basic Surgical Instrumentation—cont'd

Instrument	Use
Doyen	Grasping or occluding tissue

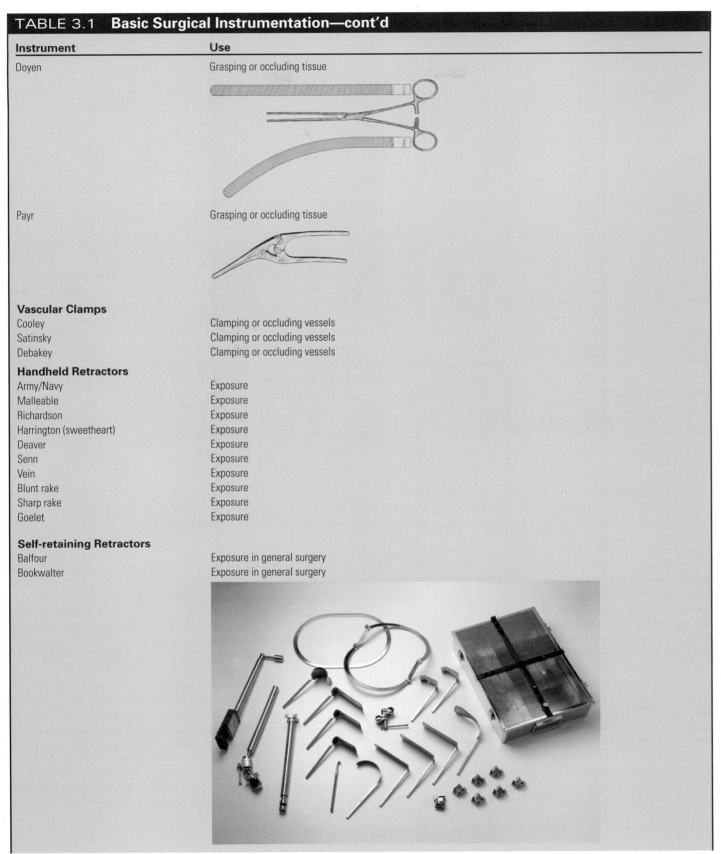

Instrument	Use
Payr	Grasping or occluding tissue

Vascular Clamps

Cooley	Clamping or occluding vessels
Satinsky	Clamping or occluding vessels
Debakey	Clamping or occluding vessels

Handheld Retractors

Army/Navy	Exposure
Malleable	Exposure
Richardson	Exposure
Harrington (sweetheart)	Exposure
Deaver	Exposure
Senn	Exposure
Vein	Exposure
Blunt rake	Exposure
Sharp rake	Exposure
Goelet	Exposure

Self-retaining Retractors

Balfour	Exposure in general surgery
Bookwalter	Exposure in general surgery

Continued

TABLE 3.1 Basic Surgical Instrumentation—cont'd

Instrument	Use
Thompson	Exposure in general and vascular surgery

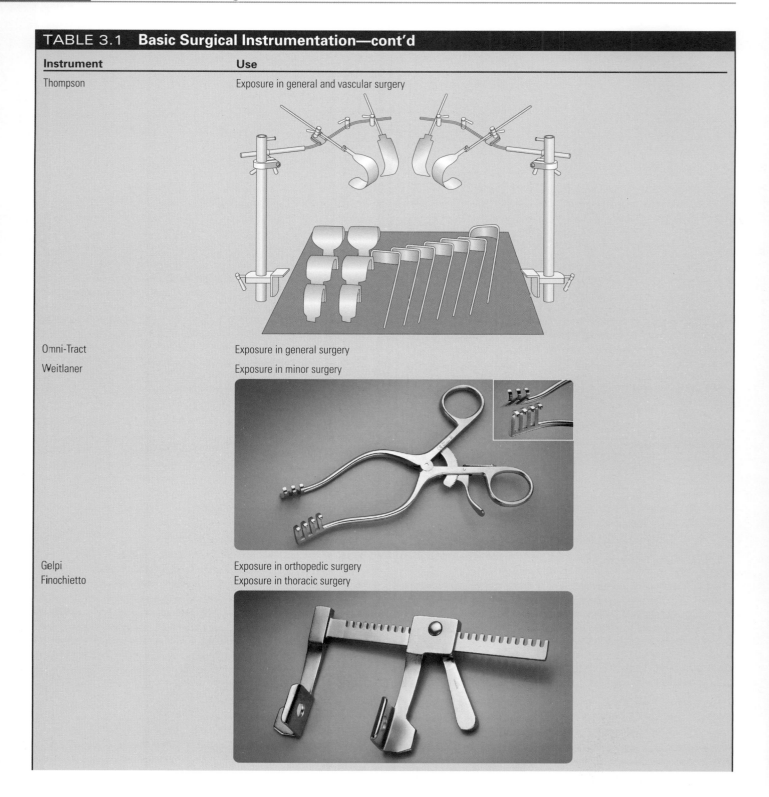

| Omni-Tract | Exposure in general surgery |
| Weitlaner | Exposure in minor surgery |

| Gelpi | Exposure in orthopedic surgery |
| Finochietto | Exposure in thoracic surgery |

TABLE 3.1 **Basic Surgical Instrumentation—cont'd**

Instrument	Use
O'Sullivan/O'Connor	Exposure in OB/GYN surgery

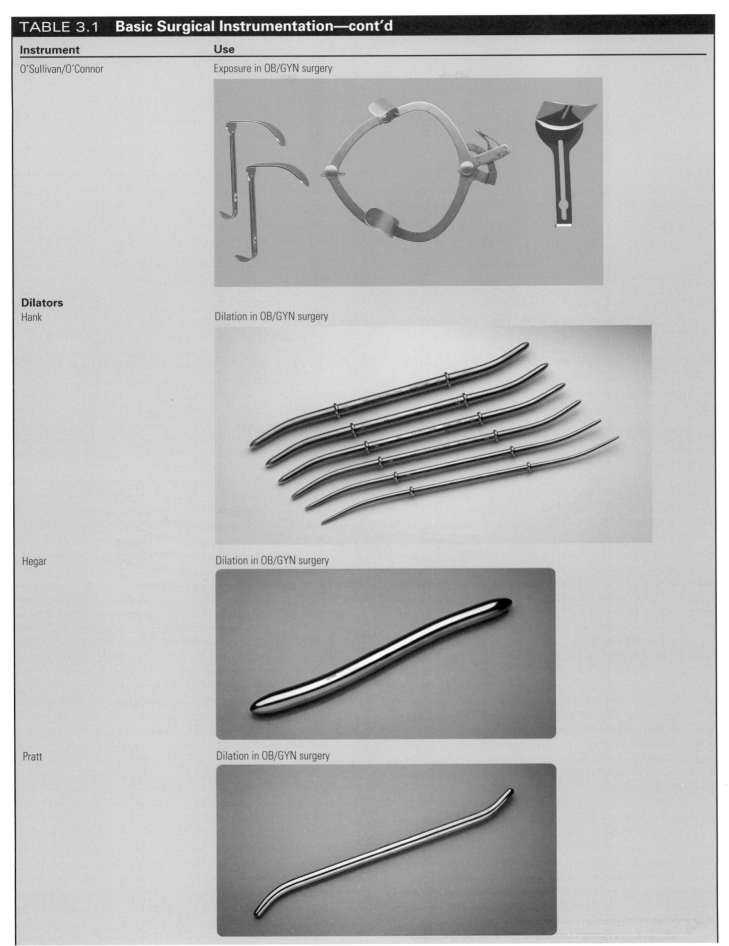

Dilators	
Hank	Dilation in OB/GYN surgery
Hegar	Dilation in OB/GYN surgery
Pratt	Dilation in OB/GYN surgery

Continued

TABLE 3.1 Basic Surgical Instrumentation—cont'd

Instrument	Use
Van Buren	Dilation in genitourinary surgery
Bakes	Dilation of common bile duct

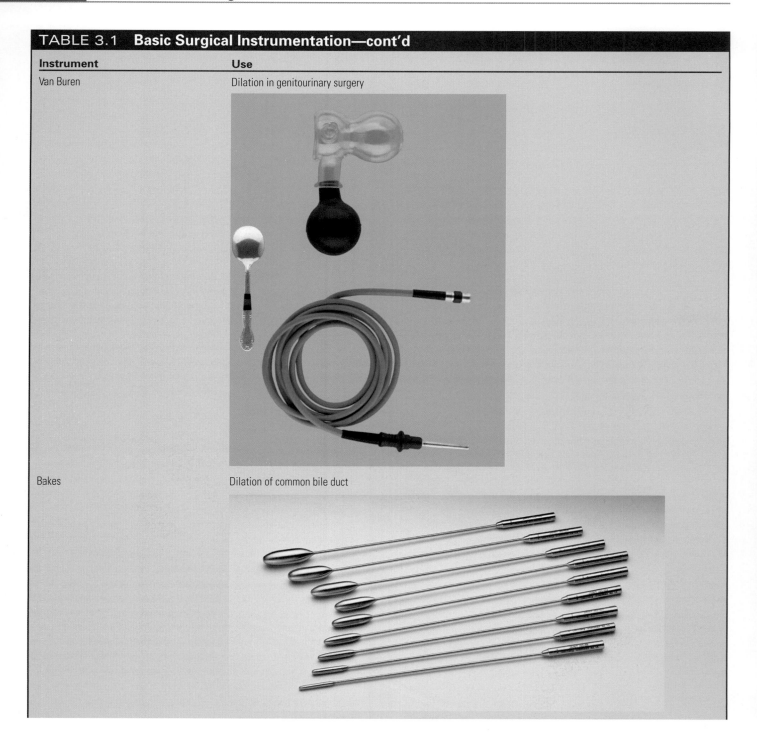

TABLE 3.1 Basic Surgical Instrumentation—cont'd

Instrument	Use
Needle Holders	
Mayo	Suturing
Webster	Suturing skin closures

Castroviejo	Suturing of vascular anastomoses
Heaney	Suturing (most commonly in GYN procedures such as vaginal and abdominal hysterectomy)

Ryder	Suturing (commonly with very small suture needles in cardiovascular, plastic, and neurosurgical procedures)

Continued

TABLE 3.1	**Basic Surgical Instrumentation—cont'd**
Instrument	**Use**
Suction Tips	
Yankhauer	Oral suctioning
Poole	Suctioning
Frazier	Suctioning
Baron	Suctioning

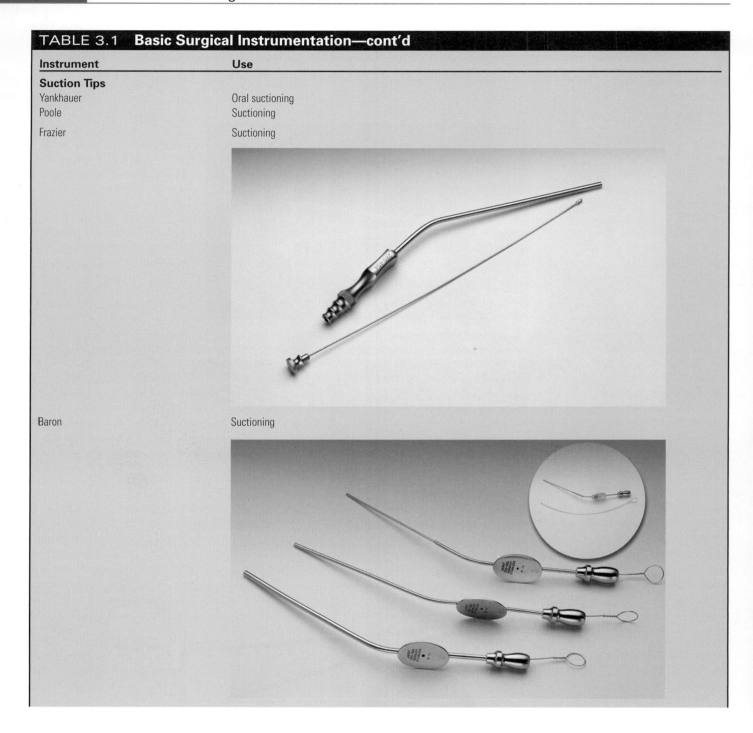

TABLE 3.1 Basic Surgical Instrumentation—cont'd

Instrument	Use

Speculums

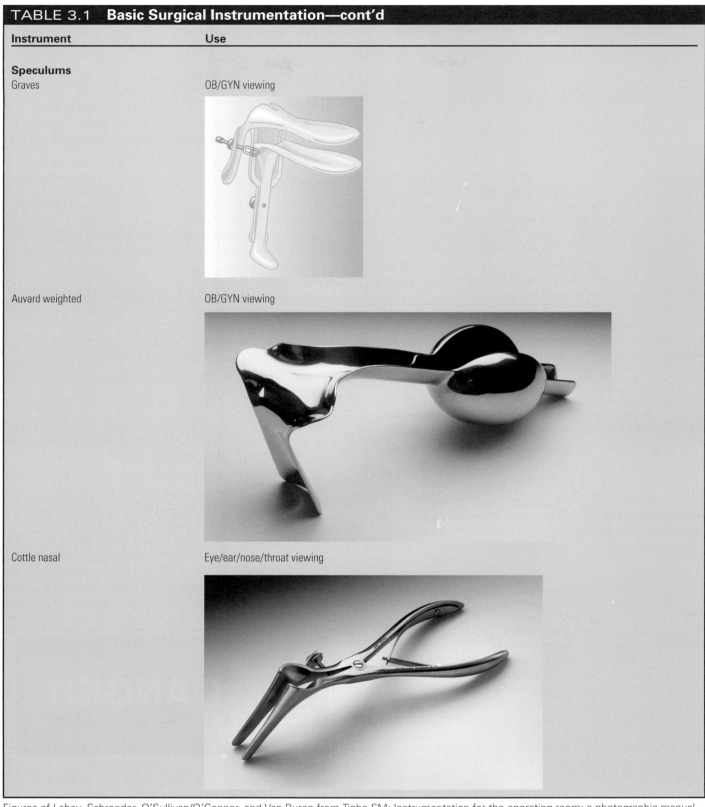

Graves — OB/GYN viewing

Auvard weighted — OB/GYN viewing

Cottle nasal — Eye/ear/nose/throat viewing

TABLE 3.2 The Vocabulary of Electricity

Term	Definition
Electricity	Free electrons flowing from one atom to another
Alternating current (AC)	Electrons flowing back and forth along a single pathway
Direct current (DC)	A current that flows in one direction, from negative to positive
Electron	A negatively charged particle that orbits an atom
Neutron	A neutral atom
Proton	A positively charged atom
Free electron	An electron that is not bound to an atom, ion, or molecule and can move freely; the basis of electricity and magnetism
Insulator	A material that inhibits the flow of electrical current
Volt	Electrical potential
Current	Flow of electrical charge, measured in amperes (amps)
Power	The rate at which work is done
Load	Device that requires electricity to perform
Switch	Device used to open or close a current

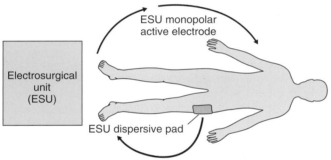

FIG. 3.4 Monopolar current path. (From Phillips N: Berry & Kohn's operating room technique, ed 13, St Louis, 2017, Elsevier.)

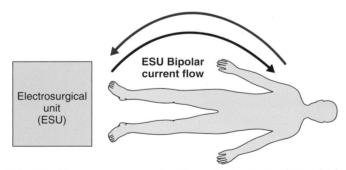

FIG. 3.5 Bipolar current path. No patient return electrode is used. (From Phillips N: Berry & Kohn's operating room technique, ed 13, St Louis, 2017, Elsevier.)

- Keep flammable anesthetics away from electrocautery electrodes.
- Give prep solutions adequate time to dry before beginning electrocautery.
- Keep a smoke evacuator with HEPA filter ready for use on the cautery plume.
- Never reuse a grounding pad.
- Never silence the alarms on the electrosurgical circuit.

Lasers

The name *laser* is an acronym for Light Amplification by Stimulated Emission of Radiation. You will encounter several types of lasers in the operating room.

CO_2 Laser

- Most frequently used laser, often in endoscopic procedures
- Uses CO_2 gas to transmit a beam that cuts and coagulates tissue
- Cannot be transmitted through fluids

ND:YAG Laser

- Laser of choice for endoscopic gastrointestinal procedures
- Uses contact delivery system
- Fiber beam absorbed by darker-pigmented tissue
- Can be transmitted through fluids

Excimer Laser

- Commonly used in radial keratoplasty (RK) and stenotic artery plaque destruction
- Uses gases and halogens as the medium

Holmium:YAG Laser

- Commonly used in arthroscopic procedures and RK
- Employs a pulsed beam

Laser Safety

- A warning sign (Fig. 3.6) should be placed every door of every room in which lasers are in use.
- All personnel in the room with a laser must use protective eyewear.
- The surgical technician in the scrub role should maintain a basin or pitcher of sterile water on field for fire prevention.
- The scrub tech should also ensure that a halon fire extinguisher, recommended for use against laser fires, is present in any operating room where a laser is being used. The halon extinguisher is chosen for its low toxicity and lack of residue.

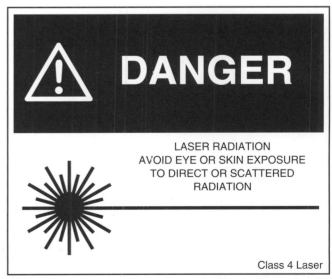

FIG. 3.6 Laser warning sign. (From Rothrock JC: Alexander's care of the patient in surgery, ed 15, St Louis, 2015, Mosby.)

- The laser should be placed on standby when not in use.
- The team should know that class C is the halon fire extinguisher appropriate for use against laser fires.
- A smoke evacuator with HEPA filter should be kept at the ready for use on the laser plume.
- Nonreflective surgical instrumentation is used to prevent beam reflection.
- Caution must be exercised when a laser is being used in head and neck area because of the flammability of anesthetics. (Anesthesia should be delivered by way of a closed system with nonflammable anesthetic gas and a nonflammable endotracheal tube [Fig. 3.7].)
- In rectal procedures, sterile water–soaked packing is placed to prevent methane gas explosion.

Robotics

The use of robotics in the operating room is expanding in scope and becoming more commonplace every day. Table 3.3 sets forth some basic terms you need to be familiar with.

The da Vinci Surgical System (Fig. 3.8), manufactured by Intuitive Surgical, is the primary robotic system in use today.

- da Vinci's EndoWrist surgical instrumentation and the elimination of hand tremor are the main selling points of this robotic system.
- The system's manipulators have 7 degrees of freedom and 90 degrees of articulation.

Imaging

Let's start our review of imaging with a little refresher on terms you're likely to encounter on your certification exam and in practice (Table 3.4).

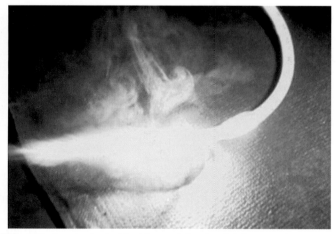

FIG. 3.7 A polyvinyl chloride endotracheal tube can become a blowtorch if ignited by a laser beam. (From Rothrock JC: Alexander's care of the patient in surgery, ed 15, St Louis, 2015. Mosby.)

TABLE 3.3 Basic Robotics Terminology

Term	Meaning
Articulation	A joint in a robotic arm
Binaural hearing	Robot's capacity to determine the origin of a sound
Manipulator	Robotic arm
Resolution	Robot's capacity to differentiate objects
Telechir	Remote-controlled manipulator

X-Rays

Fluoroscopy

- This machine produces real-time live x-ray images.
- It has a C-arm construction (Fig. 3.9).
- A sterile cover is required for intraoperative use.

Portable X-Ray Machine

- This apparatus produces single-shot X-rays.
- A sterile cover is required for use of cassettes in the sterile field.

X-Ray Safety

- Use the shortest possible exposure time to reduce radiation exposure.
- Stay at least 6 feet from the radiation .
- People in the area of the x-ray machine should wear a lead apron, lead thyroid shield, lead gloves, and leaded glasses.
- Staff should be outfitted with dosimeters to monitor their exposure to radiation.

Magnetic Resonance Imaging (MRI)

- This is the use of a magnetic field and radio waves to take pictures of structures inside the body.
- It is used for soft tissue examination.
- MRI does not involve the use of ionizing radiation.

Computed Tomography (CT)/Computed Axial Tomography (CAT) Scan

- This method involves the use of X-rays to produce "slice" images of the anatomy.
- CT is used most often to view bony structures.
- Exposure to ionizing radiation is possible.

Positron Emission Tomography (PET) Scanning

- PET scanning combines computed tomography and a radio-isotope.
- It is used for brain scanning.

Ultrasonography

- Sound waves are used for anatomy identification.
- This method does not involve the use of radiation.
- It is the imaging modality of choice for pregnant patients.

Doppler Ultrasound

- This machine produces ultrasonic waves that are bounced off circulating red blood cells to estimate blood flow through vessels (Standard **ultrasound** uses sound waves to produce images but can't show blood flow.)
- It is used to monitor heart rate and reveal the patency of blood flow.

Other Electronic Equipment

Some electronic surgical equipment (Table 3.5) doesn't fall into the aforementioned categories.

Nerve Stimulator

- This machine is used within the sterile field to identify nerve tissue for treatment or to prevent nerve injury.

Cell Saver

- This blood retrieval system allows autologous (self) collection of blood.

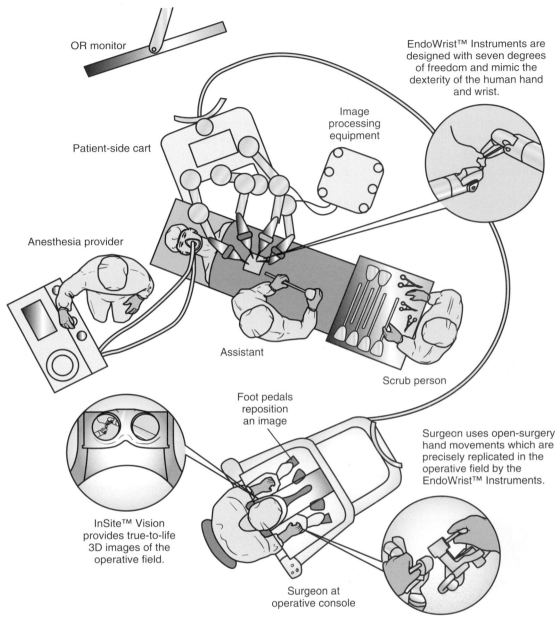

FIG. 3.8 Layout of da Vinci robotic system. (From Phillips N: Berry & Kohn's operating room technique, ed 13, St Louis, 2017, Elsevier.)

TABLE 3.4	**Basic Imaging Technology**
Term	**Meaning**
Ionizing radiation	Radiation strong enough to cause electrons to leave their atoms and become free; basis of X-ray imaging and radiation therapy
Diagnostic imaging	Any imaging performed for the purpose of diagnosing disease (as opposed to screening imaging, used to detect abnormalities)
Radiography (X-ray, C-arm)	Use of radiation to develop images of anterior and posterior anatomy

- Cell-saving is contraindicated in patients with infections or cancer.
- The cell saver is also used in patients who refuse blood transfusions, most notably members of the Jehovah's Witnesses religious sect.

DECONTAMINATION, DISINFECTION, AND STERILIZATION

Different pieces of equipment used in different ways require different methods of cleansing. There are three main categories of cleanup used to return instruments and equipment to service cleansed of debris and microorganisms (Fig. 3.11).

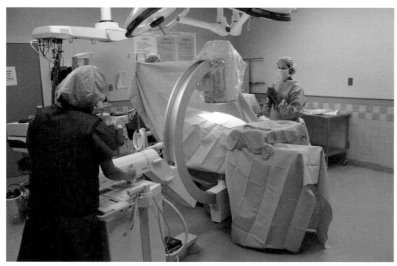

FIG. 3.9 Radiographer carefully moves a C-arm mobile fluoroscope into position in operating room. Note wrapping of image intensifier to prevent contamination of sterile field by dust from equipment. (From Ehrlich RA, Coakes DM: Patient care in radiography with an introduction to medical imaging, ed 9, St Louis, 2017, Elsevier.)

TABLE 3.5	Other Electronic Surgical Equipment.
Device	**Function**
Nerve stimulator	Used in sterile field to identify nerve tissue
Cell saver	Autologous (self) blood-retrieval system (contraindicated in patients with infection or cancer)
Harmonic scalpel (Fig. 3.10)	Ultrasonic (sound) energy to cut and coagulate tissue (no grounding pad)
CO_2 insufflator	Used to establish pneumoperitoneum (inflation of the abdominal cavity) for laparoscopic procedures
Cavitron Ultrasonic Surgical Aspirator (CUSA)	Ultrasonic (sound) energy used to emulsify and absorb tissue
Cryotherapy unit	Cold probe freezes tissue
Irrigation and aspiration unit (pulse lavage)	Powered irrigation unit used to debride wounds
Dermatome (Brown, Padgett, Reese)	Used to harvest a split-thickness skin graft
Operating microscope	Used to magnify tissue for better visualization

Decontamination

This is the process by which used equipment, medical devices, and surgical instrumentation are rendered safe for central supply personnel to handle for sterile processing.

Decontamination begins at the point of use:

- Personal protective equipment (PPE)
- Protective eyewear, gloves, gown or waterproof apron, waterproof shoe covers or boots
- Transport of soiled instrumentation in a closed cart
- Disassembly and unlocking of soiled instrumentation to permit processing

Disinfection

Destruction of microorganisms by heat or chemical means is known as disinfection. This mode of cleaning, commonly

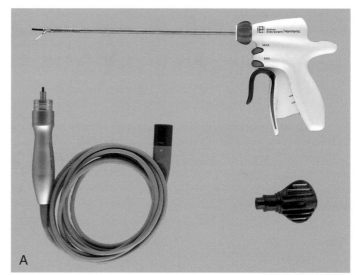

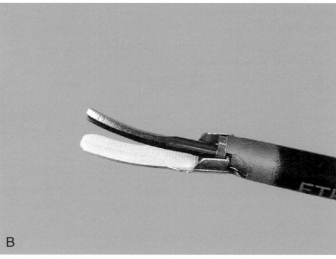

FIG. 3.10 **A,** *Top to bottom:* 1 Harmonic scalpel 5 mm, 23 cm; 1 Harmonic cord and 1 tightening key. **B,** Enlarged tip: Harmonic scalpel 5 mm with curved shears. (From Tighe SM: Instrumentation for the operating room: a photographic manual, ed 9, St Louis, 2016, Mosby.)

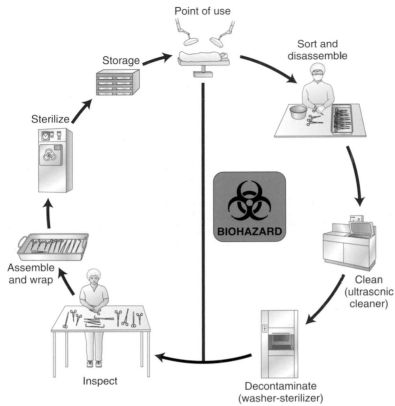

FIG. 3.11 Cycle of reprocessing, starting at the point of use. (From Fuller JK: *Surgical technology: Principles and practice,* ed 6, St Louis, 2013, Saunders.)

applied to inanimate objects, comprises several levels of thoroughness:

Cleaning

- Physical removal of gross debris (bioburden), including human bodily fluids and blood
- Accomplished with the use of an enzymatic cleaner

Low-Level Disinfection

- Involves the use of isopropyl alcohol and ethyl alcohol (in a 60%–70% dilution) on noncritical surfaces
- Achieved in **10 to 15 minutes**
- Kills several types of microorganisms:
  - Tuberculocidal
  - Bactericidal
  - Virucidal
  - Fungicidal

Intermediate Disinfection

- Involves the application of **phenol** (carbolic acid), usually diluted with tap water and used on large areas such as floors and countertops
- Achieved in **10 to 15 minutes**
- Kills several types of microorganisms:
  - **Bactericidal**
  - **Virucidal** (nonhydrophilic viruses)
  - **Fungicidal**

High-Level Disinfection

- This type of disinfection is achieved with the use of **glutaraldehyde** (sometimes sold under the brand name **Cidex**).
- It is used on surgical devices such as **rigid and flexible endoscopes** that require **immersion** in the liquid for disinfection or sterilization (discussed later in the chapter).
- For an instrument to be disinfected, it must be dry before being soaked (completely immersed) for **20 minutes** at room temperature.
- Immersion for **10 hours** achieves total sterilization.
- Glutaraldehyde kills many microorganisms:
  - **Tuberculocidal**
  - **Bactericidal** (gram-positive and -negative bugs)
  - **Virucidal**
  - **Fungicidal**
  - **Sporicidal**
- OSHA calls for the use of appropriate **ventilation** when glutaraldehyde is used.

Sterilization

This is the process by which all microorganisms, including spores, are destroyed. There are several methods of accomplishing this.

Steam Autoclaving

- The **gravity displacement cycle** is run at 15 to 17 psi and 250° F for 15 to 30 minutes.

- The **prevacuum cycle** is run at 27 psi and 270° to 276° F for 15 to 30 minutes.
- **Immediate-use steam (flash) sterilization** is conducted at 27 psi and 270° F, with a minimum processing time of 3 minutes (10 minutes for instrumentation with a lumen).

Ethylene Oxide (ETO) Gas

- A **2- to 3-hour processing time** is required.
- A **10- to 12-hour aeration cycle** is carried out in a separate aeration machine.
- This gas is flammable and a potential carcinogen, so **OSHA guidelines** for exposure must be followed.
- This is the preferred method of **sterilizing delicate scopes and cameras.**

Glutaraldehyde (Cidex)

- Sterilization is accomplished through immersion in the liquid chemical for **10 hours**; as with high-level disinfection, the instrument must be **dry** before being immersed in glutaraldehyde.
- Flushing of lumens and rinsing of items with **sterile water** is required before use.

STERRAD (Hydrogen Peroxide Plasma)

- This method involves a **low-temperature drying process.**
- One cycle takes **1 hour.**

STERIS (Peracetic Acid)

- Cycle time is **20 to 35 minutes.**
- Items processed are for **immediate use**, not wrapped and stored for later.

Quality-Assurance Methods

Biological Indicators (Guarantee Sterility of Items)

- These indicators, consisting of test tubes containing certain **bacterial strains**, challenge the efficacy of an autoclave being used for sterilization; results are documented after every run.
- *Geobacillus stearothermophilus* is used for **steam sterilizers.**
  - This indicator is run **daily or weekly.**
  - *G. stearothermophilus* is incubated for **24 hours** before a reading is recorded.
  - It is incubated at **131° to 140° F (50°–55° C).**
- *Bacillus subtilis* is used for **ethylene oxide sterilizers** and run on every load.
- **Spore strips** are processed to determine the efficacy of STERRAD and STERIS.

Chemical Indicators (Reveal Exposure to the Sterilization Process)

- Autoclave tape, used to seal sterile packaging of instrumentation trays, **changes color** upon exposure.
- Indicator strips are placed **inside** items to be processed for sterilization and change color upon exposure.

CONCLUSION

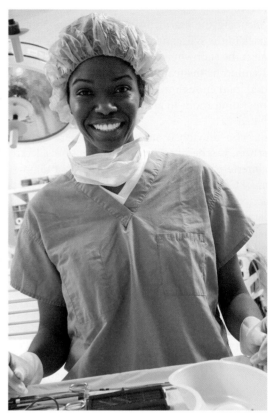

(Copyright © moodboard/Getty Images.)

Now that you've completed this review of various facets of the surgical environment, you should be ready to complete the Chapter 3 review questions. You can check your answers on the Evolve Resources site. If you feel that you need more review, make your way through the chapter again, focusing on any areas of weakness.

REVIEW QUESTIONS

1. The surgeon asks you to shut off the audible warning sounds on the ESU, saying that they're annoying and a distraction. What is the appropriate action to take?
   a. Silencing the alarm and submitting an event report to the quality department
   b. Turning up the radio so the alarm will not seem as loud and annoying to the team and relying on the lights on the unit to alert the staff when the ESU is activated
   c. Silencing the alarm, using the volume control on the back of the ESU, and relying on the lights on the unit to alert the staff when the ESU is activated
   d. Reminding the team that the alarms should be activated and loud enough to be heard above other sounds in the operating room to alert the staff when the ESU is activated

2. Zeke, who previously underwent surgery for pacemaker insertion, is scheduled for colon resection. Electrosurgery can interfere with a pacemaker's circuitry and function and create ECG artifacts. Although modern pacemakers are designed to be shielded from radiofrequency current, they are subject to interference during electrosurgery use, and certain precautions should be followed.
   1. Conducting continuous monitoring of the patient (i.e. ECG and peripheral pulse at minimum) during electrosurgery
   2. Having a defibrillator immediately available for emergencies during surgery
   3. Keeping all electrosurgical cords and cables away from the pacemaker and its leads
   4. Using bipolar electrosurgery whenever possible and using the lowest possible setting on the ESU

   What are the appropriate actions to take for patients with electrical implants during surgery in which an ESU will be used?
   a. 2, 4
   b. 1, 2, 4
   c. 1, 3, 4
   d. 1, 2, 3, 4

3. The term given to the continuous flow of air from inside the operating room outward is:
   a. Laminar air flow
   b. Negative pressure
   c. Reverse air flow
   d. Direct pressure

4. The temperature of the operating room is maintained at:
   a. 60° to 65° F
   b. 68° to 73° F
   c. 74° to 79° F
   d. 60° to 73° F

5. Who maintains the safety and operating conditions of many operating room devices?
   a. Surgical technologist
   b. Environmentalist
   c. Operating room nurse
   d. Biomedical personnel

6. All of the following areas are considered unrestricted **except** the:
   a. Family waiting room
   b. OR suite changing room
   c. Dining area
   d. Surgical suite

7. In which of these areas must the surgical technologist wear scrub attire, including complete head, nose, and mouth covering, at all times?
   a. Corridor between surgical rooms
   b. PACU
   c. Operating room
   d. Anesthesia workroom

8. The process by which used equipment, medical devices, and surgical instrumentation are rendered safe for personnel to handle is:
   a. Decontamination
   b. Sterilization
   c. Disinfection
   d. Terminal cleaning

9. The process in which microorganisms are destroyed with the use of heat or chemical means is called:
   a. Decontamination
   b. Sterilization
   c. Terminal cleaning
   d. Disinfection

10. The process by which all microorganisms, including spores, are destroyed is:
    a. Sterilization
    b. Decontamination
    c. Terminal cleaning
    d. Disinfection

11. Glutaraldehyde (Cidex) is used in surgical devices such as rigid and flexible endoscopes that require immersion for disinfection or sterilization to be achieved. For how long must these instruments be dry before being soaked or completely immersed to achieve disinfection?
    a. 30 minutes
    b. 10 hours
    c. 20 minutes
    d. 24 hours

12. Of all the methods available for sterilization, moist heat in the form of saturated steam under pressure is the most widely used and the most dependable. Steam sterilization is nontoxic, inexpensive, and rapidly microbicidal and sporicidal, and it rapidly heats and penetrates fabrics. There are recognized minimum exposure periods for sterilization of wrapped healthcare supplies. How much exposure in gravity displacement is required for sterilization of wrapped instruments?
    a. 25 minutes at 250° F
    b. 30 minutes at 250° F
    c. 35 minutes at 250° F
    d. 40 minutes at 250° F

13. The Bowie-Dick test is a:
    a. Chemical indicator for sterilization
    b. Biological indicator
    c. Indicator of water leaks
    d. Indicator of air leaks
14. Cleaning is an integral component of virtually all instrument-reprocessing guidelines. Several endoscopy and infection-control organizations have published guidelines for the proper cleaning and sterilization of flexible endoscopes, biopsy forceps, and other types of endoscopic instruments. Which type of energy is routinely used by healthcare facilities to clean surgical and dental instruments before terminal sterilization?
    a. Ultrasonic
    b. Sonic
    c. Electric
    d. Magnetic
15. Which of these statements about the washer/disinfecter or sterilizer is true?
    a. It kills vegetative and spore-bearing microorganisms.
    b. It kills spore-bearing microorganisms only.
    c. It kills vegetative microorganisms only.
    d. None of the above.
16. Alisha notices that her assigned operating room is scheduled for six laparoscopic surgeries. The hospital has only three laparoscopy sets. The turnover time between cases will be 35 minutes. How will Alisha handle the situation?
    a. By soaking all of the instrument sets in alcohol for 30 minutes
    b. By soaking the light , camera and lens in povidone-iodine (Betadine) solution for 30 minutes and washing the instruments in the washer/sterilizer.
    c. By autoclaving the instruments on a prevacuum cycle and soaking the light , camera and lens in glutaraldehyde (Cidex) for 10 minutes
    d. By autoclaving all of the instruments on a prevacuum cycle

17. PPE (personal protective equipment) consists of:
    a. Protective eyewear and shoe covers
    b. Protective eyewear, a waterproof apron, and boots
    c. Protective eyewear, gloves, and gown or waterproof apron
    d. Protective eyewear, gloves, gown or waterproof apron, and waterproof shoe covers or boots
18. Electrical cords should be inspected before surgery by:
    a. The surgical technologist
    b. The nurse anesthetist
    c. An electrician
    d. The surgeon
19. It is considered best practice to:
    a. Change a glove on recognizing that it is contaminated
    b. Not to change a glove on learning that a case is contaminated
    c. Administer additional antibiotics when it becomes evident that a case is contaminated
    d. Change a glove after recognizing that it is contaminated and informing the surgeon as well.
20. The best way to protect oneself from radiation during the use of a C-arm or other x-ray apparatus in the operating room is to:
    a. Stand behind the glass door leading to the substerile area
    b. Wearing a lead apron
    c. Wearing a lead apron and thyroid shield
    d. Standing at least 3 feet from the machine

Surgical Case Management: Surgical Microbiology and Wound Management

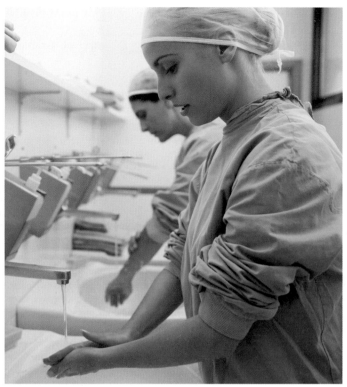

(Copyright © Wavebreakmedia Ltd/Wavebreak Media/Getty Images.)

There's much more to surgery than just the procedure itself. Cutting into living flesh, whether it's done surgically or traumatically, carries a risk of morbidity and mortality resulting from infection.

SURGICAL MICROBIOLOGY

Perhaps the greatest challenge in any surgical procedure is the prevention of infection.

Surgical site infection, or SSI, is infection occurring in the 30 days following a surgery (or, in patients receiving implants, as much as 1 year after surgery).

SSIs are not all alike. The causative organism behind an SSI depends on:
- Type of surgery
- The surgical conscience of the members of the operating room team (i.e., surgical technologist, surgeon, and surgical nurse). (The concept of surgical conscience is discussed in Chapter 6.)
- The cleanliness of the surgical environment
- The origin of the microorganism (e.g., the resident flora)
- The health of the patient (e.g., immune defenses)

Centers for Disease Control and Prevention guidelines for the prevention of SSIs emphasize the importance of good patient preparation, aseptic practice, and attention to surgical technique; antimicrobial prophylaxis is also indicated in specific circumstances.

Characteristics of Bacteria

A solid understanding of cells—their types, structures, and means of multiplication and metabolism—is crucial for the surgical technologist, because it will help you determine the level and means of cleansing and type of pharmacology needed to eliminate a particular microorganism to help prevent SSIs.

Eukaryotes and Prokaryotes

Living cells are divided into two groups (Fig. 4.1):
- Eukaryotic cells make up animals and plants. Each eukaryotic cell has a nucleus and mitochondria, among other structures.
- A prokaryotic cell has no nucleus, mitochondria, or most of the other cell structures seen in eukaryotes. All bacteria are prokaryotes.

Gram Staining

One common means of differentiating cells is how they react to a process called Gram staining (Fig. 4.2). In this method of detecting bacteria, a specimen is treated first with crystal violet stain and then, to bind the crystal violet, iodide. The specimen is then washed with ethanol and finally counterstained with a dye called safranin. (Fig. 4.3 depicts a specimen in which one organism stained gram-positive.)

Gram-Positive Bacteria

On a positive Gram stain, bacteria retain the crystal violet after being treated with iodide and washed with ethanol, taking on

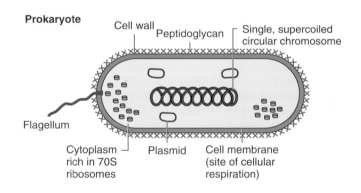

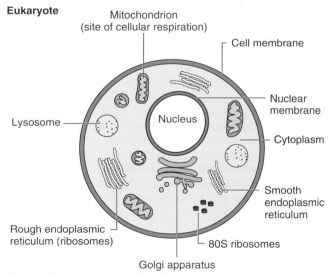

FIG. 4.1 Major features of prokaryotes and eukaryotes. (From Murray PR, Rosenthal KS, Pfaller MA: Medical microbiology, ed 8, Philadelphia, 2016, Elsevier.)

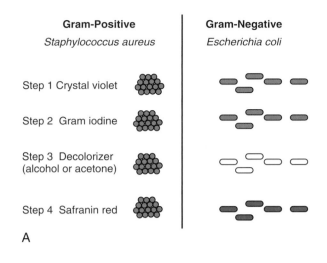

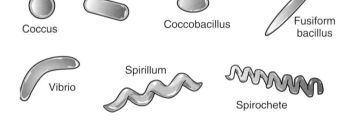

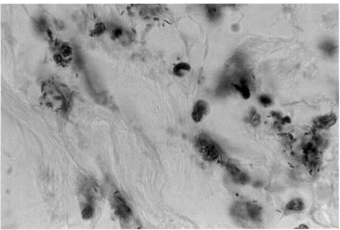

FIG. 4.2 Gram-stain morphology of bacteria. **A,** The crystal violet of Gram stain is precipitated by Gram iodine and is trapped in the thick peptidoglycan layer in gram-positive bacteria. The decolorizer disperses the gram-negative outer membrane and washes the crystal violet from the thin layer of peptidoglycan. Gram-negative bacteria are visualized by the red counterstain. **B,** Bacterial morphologies. (From Murray PR, Rosenthal KS, Pfaller MA: Medical microbiology, ed 8, Philadelphia, 2016, Elsevier.)

FIG. 4.3 Gram stain reveals a *Mycobacterium* pathogen (the purple rod-shaped bacilli) in a skin-derived tissue sample. (Courtesy Centers for Disease Control and Prevention/Dr. Roger Feldman.)

a purple coloration. There are three types of gram-positive bacteria:

- **Aerobic** organisms require oxygen for survival. Examples include:
  - *Bacillus anthracis*, which causes anthrax
  - Corynebacterium diphtheriae, the cause of diphtheria
  - *Listeria monocytogenes*, which causes listeriosis, a serious infection usually spread in contaminated food
  - *Lactobacillus* species, "friendly" bacteria that normally live in our digestive, urinary, and genital tracts without causing disease
- **Anaerobic** organisms do not need oxygen to survive. Examples include:
  - *Clostridium perfringens*, the most common cause of gas gangrene
  - *Clostridium botulinum*, a spore-forming, motile bacterium that produces the neurotoxin botulinum; grows on food and produces toxins that, when ingested, cause paralysis
  - *Clostridium difficile*, which causes diarrhea and more serious intestinal conditions such as colitis
- **Facultative anaerobic** organisms can use oxygen but also use anaerobic methods of energy production, making them able to survive in just about any environment. Examples include:
  - *Enterococcus* species, which cause a variety of illnesses, including urinary tract infections, bacteremia, endocarditis, and meningitis.
  - *Staphylococcus aureus*, which is responsible for several types of disorders and illnesses:
    - Skin infection: small benign boils, folliculitis, impetigo, cellulitis, and more severe, invasive soft-tissue infections
    - Bacteremia: presence of bacteria in the bloodstream, resulting in infection of various organs that can cause infective endocarditis, septic arthritis, and osteomyelitis
  - *Staphylococcus epidermis*, a pathogen of particular concern for people with catheters or other surgical implants because it is known to form biofilms on such devices
  - *Streptococcus agalactiae*, found in the human gastrointestinal flora and in the female urogenital tract and rectum; causes postpartum infection and is the most common cause of neonatal sepsis
  - *Streptococcus mutans*, which is found in the human oral cavity and is a major contributor to tooth decay
  - *Streptococcus pneumonia*, which causes community-acquired pneumonia (CAP), bacterial meningitis, bacteremia, and otitis media, as well as sinusitis, septic arthritis, osteomyelitis, peritonitis, and endocarditis
  - *Streptococcus pyogenes*, which causes acute pharyngitis, toxic shock syndrome (TSS), and life-threatening skin and soft tissue infections, especially necrotizing fasciitis

Gram-Negative Bacteria

Bacteria that do not retain crystal violet after being treated with iodide and washed with ethanol are considered gram-negative.

All gram-negative bacteria take up the safranin counterstain, which turns them hot pink or red. There are also three kinds of gram-negative bacteria:

- **Aerobic gram-negative** organisms include:
  - *Bordetella pertussis*, which causes pertussis, better known as whooping cough
  - *Neisseria gonorrhoeae*, which causes the sexually transmitted disease gonorrhea
  - *Neisseria meningitides*, which causes meningococcal disease
  - *Moraxella catarrhalis*, a common cause of otitis media in infants and children, responbsible for 15% to 20% of acute otitis media episodes
  - *Acinebacter* species, the cause of many hospital-acquired (nosocomial) infections such as bacteremia, urinary tract infection (UTI), secondary meningitis, infective endocarditis, and wound and burn infections
  - *Bartonella* species, which causes cat scratch disease (CSD), bacillary angiomatosis (BA), and other infections in patients with HIV infection, as well as endocarditis
  - *Legionella pneumophila*, which causes a serious type of pneumonia (lung infection) called Legionnaires' disease
  - *Pseudomonas aeruginosa*, "blue-green pus bacteria," a species that opportunistically infects people, especially those who are immunocompromised
  - *Helicobacter pylori*, which causes ulcers in the lining of stomach and the upper part of the small intestine
  - *Rickettsia rickettsii*, the cause of Rocky Mountain spotted fever (RMSF), which is transmitted to humans through the bites of infected tick species
  - *Campylobacter jejuni*, the most common cause of community-acquired inflammatory enteritis, which produces an inflammatory, bloody diarrhea or dysentery syndrome
  - *Treponema pallidum*, the cause of syphilis, pinta, bejel, and yaws, is sexually transmitted
- **Anaerobic gram-negative** bacteria include:
  - *Bacteroides fragilis*, responsible for 90% of anaerobic peritoneal infections but also causes bacteremia associated with intraabdominal infections, peritonitis and abscesses following rupture of viscus, and subcutaneous abscesses or burns near the anus
  - *Porphyromonas gingivalis*, which causes chronic adult periodontitis
- **Facultative anaerobic gram-negative** organisms include:
  - *Haemophilus influenzae*, which causes severe illnesses such as meningitis (but can be prevented from infecting people with a vaccine)
  - *Gardnerella vaginalis*, the cause of an infection of the female genital tract called vaginosis, characterized by a gray or yellow discharge with a "fishy" odor
  - *Escherichia coli*, most of whose strains are largely harmless but, in some cases, can cause serious food poisoning in their hosts, occasionally necessitating food recalls because of contamination

- *Klebsiella pneumoniae*, which causes variant pneumonia, typically in the form of bronchopneumonia and also bronchitis
- *Salmonella enterica*, which causes salmonellosis, resulting in diarrhea, fever, vomiting, and abdominal cramps 12 to 72 hours after infection
- *Salmonella typhi*, the cause of typhoid fever
- *Vibrio cholerae*, which secretes cholera toxin, a protein that causes profuse watery diarrhea known as "rice-water stool"
- *Proteus* species, which are common causes of UTI in patients who must wear urinary catheters for long periods

Simple Staining

In this type of stain, a single dye is used to detect bacteria. One example is methylene blue (Fig. 4.4), which is retained by certain types of bacteria after the stained specimen is washed with water.

Acid-Fast Staining

In this type of staining, a red dye called carbol fuchsin is washed over the specimen, after which a solution containing hydrochloric acid is applied, followed by a dye in a contrasting color (generally methylene blue). Acid-fast bacteria remain red; non–acid-fast bacteria lose the red stain and take on the blue one. This method is used to detect, among other microbes, those of the *Mycobacterium* genus, which stain blue (Fig. 4.5).

Commonly Tested Microorganisms

Now that you've had a chance to review the basics of bacteria, let's talk about the microorganisms you're most likely to encounter on a certification exam (Table 4.1).

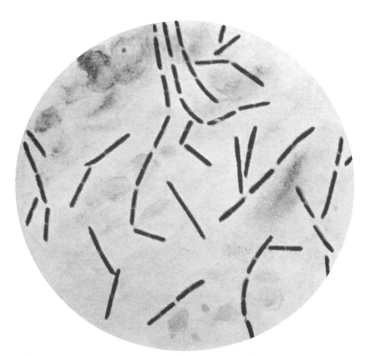

FIG. 4.4 This illustration depicts a photomicrographic view of a methylene blue–stained culture specimen revealing the presence of numerous *Clostridium septicum* bacteria. (Courtesy Centers for Disease Control and Prevention.)

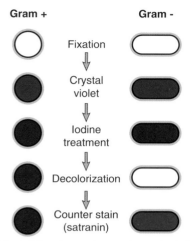

FIG. 4.5 Acid-fast *Mycobacterium tuberculosis* bacillus is visible within granuloma.

DISINFECTION AND STERILIZATION

A solid understanding of the various classifications of microorganisms gives you a basis for determining which procedures and chemicals to use in prepping surgical patients (e.g., showering with an antiseptic soap or solution), instrument sterilization (e.g., autoclaving), equipment, and the physical environment (e.g., temperature, humidity, laminar flow) to prevent SSI.

Disinfection

In the process of disinfection, nearly all microorganisms on inanimate surfaces (clothing, hard surfaces) and/or wounds are destroyed through the use of chemicals or other physical agents (Fig. 4.6). (Keep in mind, however, that disinfection doesn't destroy spore-bearing microorganisms.)

TABLE 4.1	Microorganisms Commonly Associated with SSI		
Microorganism	**Classification**	**Common Locations**	**Infection/Symptoms**
Staphylococcus aureus	Gram-positive facultative anaerobe	Skin Hair Upper respiratory tract	Surgical sites Encocarditis Osteomyelitis Toxic shock syndrome
Staphylococcus epidermis	Gram-positive facultative anaerobe	Skin Mucous membranes (e.g., mouth, nose, opening of anus)	Common on urinary catheters and implants Endocarditis
Streptococcus pneumoniae	Gram-positive facultative anaerobe	Upper respiratory tract (including throat and nasal passages)	Bacteremia Otitis media Meningitis Best known for causing pneumonia
Streptococcus pyogenes	Gram-positive – facultative anaerobe (β-hemolytic group A *Streptococcus*)	Found in carrier state in: Anus Vagina Skin Pharynx	Necrotizing fasciitis ("flesh- eating bacteria") Scarlet fever Tonsillitis Strep throat Rheumatic fever
Streptococcus mutans	Gram-positive facultative anaerobe	Mouth	Leading cause of dental caries (tooth decay)
Enterococcus species	Gram-positive–facultative anaerobic	Intestine	Urinary tract infection Bacteremia Wound infections Endocarditis
Escherichia coli	Gram-negative–facultative anaerobic	Large intestine (aids digestion, absorption, vitamin K production)	UTI Food poisoning
Pseudomonas aeruginosa	Gram-negative–aerobic	Skin	Hospital patients, especially those on ventilators, with devices such as catheters, or with surgical or burn wounds; risk for life-threatening infection
Clostridium perfringens	Gram-positive anaerobic	Normal intestinal flora	Responsible for many gastrointestinal illnesses, ranging from mild enterotoxemia to fatal gas gangrene
Clostridium difficile	Gram-positive anaerobic	Intestine	Patients taking antibiotics; symptoms include: Watery diarrhea Fever Loss of appetite Nausea Pseudomembranous colitis
Prion (proteinaceous infectious particle)	Virus	May be transmitted by consumption of infected beef Spreads in grafts of dura mater (tissue covering the brain), donated corneas, inadequately sterilized brain electrodes, contaminated growth hormone from cadaver pituitaries	Believed to cause Creutzfeldt-Jakob disease (CJD) (only way to confirm CJD is brain biopsy or autopsy)

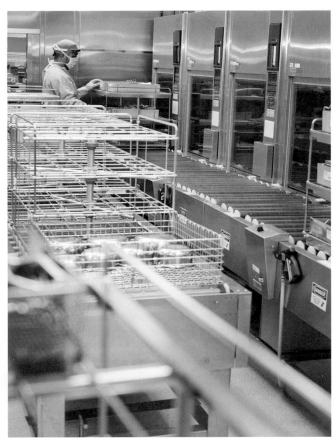

FIG. 4.6 Processing area and washer-sterilizer or decontaminator used to process soiled instruments and equipment so that personnel can handle them for assembly, wrapping, and storage. (Courtesy STERIS Corporation 2008. All rights reserved.)

There is a hierarchy of disinfection methods, which we'll review here.

Cleaning

- Physical removal of gross debris (bioburden) and human bodily fluids, including blood
- Mainly achieved with the use of soap and water

Low-Level Disinfection

- Isopropyl alcohol and ethyl alcohol (in a 60%–70% dilution)
- Used on noncritical surfaces (e.g., devices that come into contact with skin, such as a pneumatic tourniquet or pulse oximeter or the operating table) surfaces
- Achieves disinfection in 10 to 15 minutes
  - Tuberculocidal
  - Bactericidal
  - Virucidal
  - Fungicidal

Intermediate Disinfection

- Phenol (carbolic acid), usually diluted with tap water
- Used to disinfect large areas such as floors and countertops
- Achieves disinfection in 10 to 15 minutes
  - Bactericidal
  - Virucidal (non-hydrophilic viruses)
  - Fungicidal

High-Level Disinfection

- Activated glutaraldehyde (one brand name is Cidex)
- Used on surgical devices such as rigid and flexible endoscopes that requires immersion for disinfection or sterilization
- For **disinfection**, instruments must be dry before being soaked or immersed for **20 minutes** at room temperature
- For **sterilization**, instruments must be dry before being soaked or immersed for **10 hours** at room temperature
  - Tuberculocidal
  - Bactericidal (gram-positive and -negative organisms)
  - Virucidal
  - Fungicidal
  - Sporicidal

Sterilization

Steam Sterilization

See Fig. 4.7.
- Two types:
  - **Gravity displacement**
  - **Prevacuum autoclave**
- **Four parameters** of steam sterilization:
  - The **ideal type of steam** for sterilization is dry saturated steam and entrained water (dryness fraction ≥ 97%).
  - **Pressure** serves as a means of achieving the high temperatures necessary to quickly kill microorganisms.
  - Specific **temperatures** must be achieved to ensure the destruction of microorganisms (microbicidal activity). The two common steam-sterilizing temperatures are 121° C (250° F) and 132° C (270° F). These temperatures (and other high temperatures) must be maintained for a set time to kill microorganisms.
  - The recognized minimum exposure **time** for sterilization of wrapped healthcare supplies is 30 minutes at 121° C (250° F) in a gravity-displacement sterilizer or 4 minutes at 132° C (270° C) in a prevacuum sterilizer (Tables 4.2, 4.3, and 4.4).
- There are **three important phases** in both types of steam sterilization:
  - In **conditioning** (gravity-displacement autoclave) and **preconditioning** (prevacuum autoclave), the air is removed and replaced with steam.
  - Items must remain in the autoclave chamber for a particular **exposure time** (i.e., a specific duration and temperature).
  - During **drying time** (a.k.a. exhaust time), the pressure in the chamber is reduced and loads are exposed to cool air before being placed on the shelf.

Biological Indicators

These devices are the only type of monitor that can confirm that an instrument has been rendered sterile.
- Steam sterilization–*Geobacillus stearothermophilus*
  - The test pack is placed in the area of the sterilizer that is most difficult for the sterilant to reach. This represents the coldest area of the sterilizer, where air entrapment is most likely. **The coldest point is on the bottom front of the sterilization cart,** over the chamber drain.
  - If the liquid remains red after incubation (after 24 hours, incubated at 131°–140°F [50°–55°]) it means that the spores have been destroyed (negative finding).

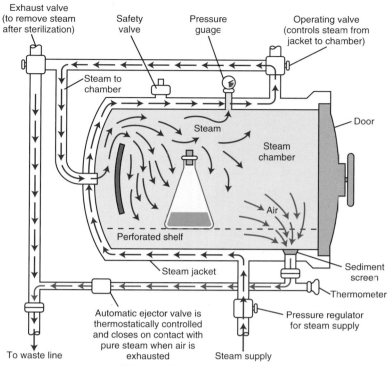

FIG. 4.7 Steam sterilization.

TABLE 4.2 Cycle Times for Gravity-Displacement Steam Sterilization

Item	Exposure Time at 250° F (121° C)	Minimum Drying Time	Exposure Time at 270° F (132° C)	Minimum Drying Time	Exposure Time at 275° F (135° C)*	Minimum Drying Time*
Wrapped instruments	30 min	15 to 30 min	15 min	15 to 30 min	10 min	30 min
Textile packs	30 min	25 min	25 min min	15 min	10 min	30 min
Wrapped utensils	30 min	30 min	15 min	15 to 30 min	10 min	10 min

*From AORN, *Perioperative standards and recommended practices, 2011 edition*. Denver, 2011, AORN.
From Rutala W, Weber D, and the Healthcare Infection Control Practices Advisory Committee (HICPAC), Atlanta, 2008, Centers for Disease Control and Prevention.

TABLE 4.3 Cycle Times for Dynamic Air Removal (Prevacuum) Steam Sterilization

Item	Exposure Time at 250° F (121° C)	Minimum Drying Time	Exposure Time at 270° F (132° C)	Minimum Drying Time	Exposure Time at 275° F (135° C)*	Minimum Drying Time*
Wrapped instruments	NA		4 min	15 to 30 min	3 min	16 min
Textile packs	NA		4 min	5 to 20 min	3 min	3 min
Wrapped utensils	NA		4 min	20 min	3 min	16 min

From Rutala W, Weber D, and the Healthcare Infection Control Practices Advisory Committee (HICPAC), Atlanta, 2008, Centers for Disease Control and Prevention.
Note: Exposure and drying times for enclosed rigid sterilization containers are specified by the manufacturer and vary according to design. Always check manufacturer's specifications for sterilization.
*From AORN, Perioperative standards and recommended practices, 2011 edition. Denver, 2011, AORN.

TABLE 4.4 Flash Steam Sterilizer (for Immediate Use) Parameters

Type of Sterilizer	Load	Temperature	Exposure Time
Gravity displacement	Metal instruments (nonporous, without lumens) only	270° to 275° F (132° to 135° C)	270° to 275° F (132° to 135° C)
	Porous items with lumens; complex power instruments (always consult manufacturer)	270° to 275° F (132° to 135° C)	10 min
Dynamic (prevacuum)	Metal instruments (non porous without lumens)	270° to 275° F (132° to 135° C)	4 min
Pressure pulse/steam flush	Nonporous /mixed porous and nonporous	270° to 275° F (132° to 135° C)	4 min

From Rutala W, Weber D, and the Healthcare Infection Control Practices Advisory Committee (HICPAC), Atlanta, 2008, Centers for Disease Control and Prevention.
Note: Exposure and for enclosed rigid sterilization containers are specified by the manufacturer and vary according to design. Always check manufacturer's specifications for sterilization using these systems.

- If the liquid turns yellow after incubation (after 24 hours, incubated at 131°–140°F [50° 55°]), spores have not been destroyed (positive finding) and sterilization has not been achieved. Loads are considered nonsterile.
- Ethylene oxide (EtO) and hydrogen peroxide gas plasma (Sterrad)–*Bacillus atrophaeus*
  - The test pack is placed in the **center** of the load because it is the most difficult place for the EtO to reach.
  - It is incubated for **48 hours**, although it is possible to read indicators after 24 hours. The pack is incubated at **95° to 98.6°F (30.5°–37°C).**
  - The use of EtO has been **discontinued** in many hospital because of the threat that the chemical poses to the **ozone layer** and because it is now known to be a **human carcinogen.**
  - **Sterrad**, which is safer, replaces EtO. The light-blue indicator tape turns **light pink** when exposed to hydrogen peroxide in plasma form.

WOUNDS

Surgery involves the creation of wounds or, in many cases, the treatment of wounds inflicted in various ways, all of which must then be encouraged to heal. We have several ways of categorizing patients' wounds—by their origin, by their degree of contamination, and by their extent of healing—and ways of closing wounds to ensure good healing.

Wound Classification

Classification by Wound Origin

Surgical Wounds

These wounds are made intentionally by a physician.

- Incisional wounds are cuts into intact skin that are made for the purpose for exposing underlying structures and growths (e.g., for pathology study).
- Excisional wounds are created by the surgeon to permit him or her to cut out (excise) diseased or damaged tissue.

Traumatic Wounds

Such wounds take two forms:

- Closed wounds are marked by underlying tissue damage even after the wound is closed by the surgeon.
- Open wounds (see Fig. 4.8 for an example) are open to the surrounding environment. There are several types:
  - Simple wounds involve compromise of skin integrity, but there is no loss of tissue and no foreign body is retained.
  - In complicated wounds, skin integrity is compromised; there is tissue loss, and a foreign body is present.
  - A clean wound's edges can be approximated and heal by primary intention (discussed later in this section). Examples include incisions made during appendectomy or breast biopsy.
  - The "contaminated" designation is applied when a dirty object comes into contact with the compromised tissue, leading to infection. Debridement is the preferred means of removing infected tissue, after which the wound is irrigated and allowed to heal by secondary (tertiary) intention.

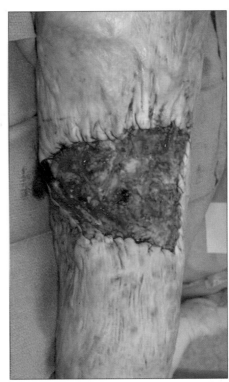

FIG. 4.8 An open wound measuring 10 cm × 7 cm resulting from a scar and ulcer excision. (From Herndon DN: *Total burn care*, ed 4, Edinburgh, 2012, Saunders.)

Chronic

Chronic wounds originate from multiple causes, but they all take time to form. Examples include:

- Pressure sores (ischemic ulcer, decubitus ulcer), result from long periods of pressure on the skin, often over a bony prominence.
- Venous ulcers occur when varicose veins go untreated, after sclerotherapy, or as a result of chronic venous insufficiency.
- Diabetic foot ulcers occur when full-thickness penetration of the dermis of the foot takes place in a person with diabetes.
- Untreated surgical site infections result from contamination of a surgical wound at the time of surgery.

Classification by Degree of Contamination

Class I: Clean

- No break in sterile technique
- Examples: coronary artery bypass grafting (CABG), craniotomy

Class II: Clean Contaminated

- Minor break in sterile technique
- Examples: controlled entry to the aerodigestive or genitourinary tract

Class III: Contaminated

- Major break in sterile technique
- Examples: open fractures, colon resection with gross spillage, stab and gunshot wounds

Class IV: Dirty

- Major break in sterile technique
- Microbial contamination before procedure
- Example: open traumatic wound more than 4 hours old

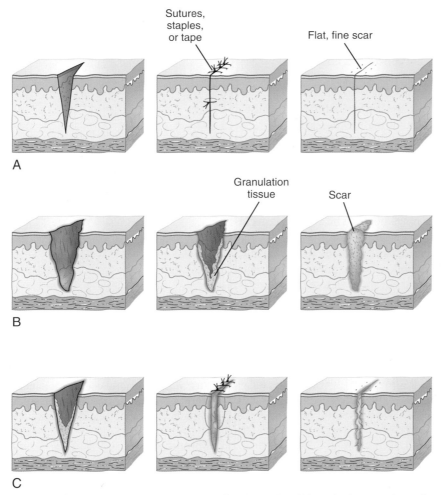

FIG. 4.9 Process of wound healing. **A,** Healing by first intention. Wound edges are brought together with sutures, staples or tape. **B,** Healing by second intention. The wound is left open because of infection that would quickly dissolve suture materials and cause further tissue reaction. The wound heals from the bottom up by continuous laying of granulation tissue. **C,** Healing by third intention. Infection is no longer present in a previously open wound, which is closed now with sutures. (From Fuller JK: *Surgical technology: Principles and practice,* ed 6, St Louis, 2013, Saunders.)

Classification by Degree of Wound Healing

See Fig. 4.9.

Primary Intention (Union, First Intention)

Phase I: Lag (Inflammatory Response)
- This initial phase begins **immediately** and lasts **3 to 5 days.**
- Signs and symptoms include heat, redness, swelling, pain, and loss of function.
- The second line of defense manifests next:
  - **Phagocytosis** is started by neutrophils and macrophages.
  - Non-epithelial tissues are reconstructed by **fibroblasts** in deeper tissue.
  - Closure of wound surfaces is made by **basal cells** that move across skin edges.

Phase II: Proliferation
- This phase begins on **day 3** after surgery and lasts **up to 20 days.**
- Wound edges are bridged by abundant **fibroblasts**, which secrete **collagen** and form fibers to gain tensile strength (up to 30%): **scar tissue.**

- On days 5 through 8, new **capillaries** form.
- On day 10, **lymphatic networks** form.

Phase III: Maturation (Differentiation)
- This phase begins on **day 14** after surgery and lasts **up to 12 months.**
- Wound contraction (lasting **21 days**) is caused by dermal and subcutaneous **myofibroblasts.**
- The scar tissue is **pale** as a result of increased collagen density and cessation of blood vessel development.
- The result is a **cicatrix**, the contracted white mature surface of a scar.

Secondary Intention (Granulation)

- This is typical when primary intention has failed.
- It is common in **large wounds or postoperative SSIs** in which infection has damaged the suture.
- The ideal treatment is removal of damaged or necrotic tissue (**debridement**).
- The wound is left open to heal from inner to outer surface (**bottom to top**).
- Granulation tissue forms:

- Soft, pink, fleshy projections consist of many capillaries surrounded by fibrous collagen.
- It forms during the healing process in a wound that does not heal by primary intention.
- Overgrowth of granulation tissue results in the growth of granulation tissue, or "proud flesh," above the skin.
- The name is taken from the Latin *granulum*, "little grain."

Tertiary Intention (Third Intention or Delayed Primary Closure)

- Primary closure of a surgical wound is delayed for several days after injury.
- This is done when a wound is initially too contaminated to be closed.

Vacuum Assisted Closure (V.A.C.; Negative-Pressure Wound Healing)

- This is a trademarked name for a system that uses the **controlled negative pressure** of a vacuum to promote healing of certain wound types.
- Wound edges are made **airtight** with the use of foam and a dressing.
- A tube is placed in the wound and connected to a canister that creates a **vacuum.**
- The vacuum **sucks** infectious materials and other fluids from the wound.

WOUND-CLOSURE DEVICES

There are several more ways, besides use of the aforementioned negative-pressure wound healing device, to close a wound (Fig. 4.10).

Sutures

A thorough knowledge of wound classification will help you choose the material for surgical wound closure and optimal healing.

Suture material is foreign to the body; the body's immune system reacts to suture and tries to destroy it. A high degree of reactivity manifests as inflammation, discomfort, delayed healing, failure to heal, and, sometimes, infection.

- Monofilament (single-strand) suture
  - This type of suture may be absorbable or non-absorbable.
  - It has low capillarity.
  - Low capillarity means that it is preferred when the risk of infection is high.
- Multifilament (multiple-strand) suture
  - This type of suture may be absorbable or non-absorbable.
  - In the presence of pathogenic bacteria, multifilament suture may draw more bacteria into a wound by way of capillarity, causing the suture to retain and spread infection within its fibers. For this reason, it is not used to close infected wounds.
  - Multifilament suture must **not** be used in the handling of diseased or infected tissue during surgery:
    - Necrotizing fasciitis
    - Abscesses
    - Removal of cancerous tissue

Bridges

These plastic devices are used to span an incision and allow retention sutures to be tightened without injuring the skin at the suture entry site (Fig. 4.11).

Bolsters

Non-latex plastic bolsters are used in various ways to reduce the strain of any temporary suture on tissue during surgery.

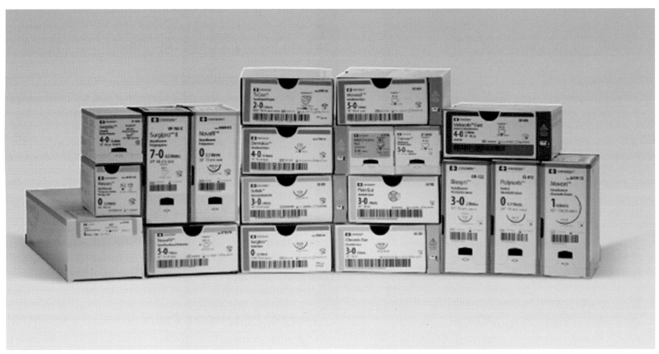

FIG. 4.10 Assorted sutures. (All rights reserved. Used with the permission of Medtronic.)

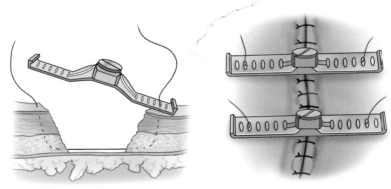

FIG. 4.11 Surgical bridge.

Bolsters may be chosen instead of bridges when retention sutures are used.
- The retention suture is threaded through the bolster
- The retention suture is then tied.
- The bolster works like a bridge, allowing the suture to be tied without injuring the skin at the suture entry site.

Skin Closure Tape

This nylon or polypropylene material is used to reinforce subcuticular (beneath-the-skin) wound closures.

Staples

These small stainless steel fasteners are used to approximate the skin edges during wound closure.

THE SURGICAL COUNT

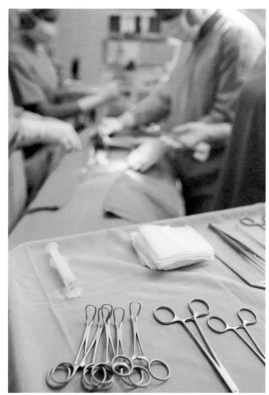

Specific items opened for a surgical procedure are counted before, during, and after the surgery in a precise way to prevent their loss in the patient. Retained surgical items (**RSI**) during surgery have safety, legal, and financial consequences.

Any item that can be retained in the surgical wound is included in the **count**. This includes sutures, surgical sponges, sharps, instruments, instrument parts, retraction devices (e.g., umbilical tapes, elastic vessel loops), instrument bolsters, suture reels, and any other small items used on the sterile field.

Retained surgical items continue to be among the most common sentinel events contributing to patient harm. A retained item can cause pain, infection, perforation of an organ, obstruction, and scarring. Repeat surgery for a retained item causes trauma, a longer recovery period, and additional expense. Severe infection or injury may result in death. Loss of an item is a sentinel event that may result in a negligence charge against any member of the surgical team.

Research shows that this event is often caused by not following established procedure. Excessive noise, lack of organization by the scrub, and pressure to hurry through procedures were found to be the features of an operative environment incompatible with correct counts. The study also identified poor communication among surgical team members as a cause of poor counting and patient risk.

Responsibility for the Count

Healthcare facilities create and enforce policies on the methodology or procedure for counts and appropriate documentation. The law does not state how counts are taken or who is to take them. The law does state that items not intended to remain in the patient must be removed before the wound is closed. All team members are responsible for ensuring that no items are left in a patient. The scrubbed technologist or nurse and circulator normally perform the count together. In turn, they report the count to the surgeon, whether it is correct or incorrect. Action taken to resolve an incorrect count is then the entire team's responsibility. During surgery, the scrubbed technologist should know at all times how many sponges, instruments, and other items are inside the patient and the location of counted items on the back table and Mayo stand.

When to Perform the Count

In general, counts are performed on all surgical or invasive procedures. Anyone on the surgical team may request a count at any time.

The healthcare facility determines policy for counting instruments, sharps, and miscellaneous items. All sponges are counted at the following times:

1. Before surgery begins to establish a baseline count and verify that the manufacturer's count is correct
2. Any time new sponges or other soft goods are added to the sterile setup (the newly added sponges are counted during distribution)
3. Before closure of any body cavity or cavity within a cavity, such as a hollow organ
4. At the start of wound closure
5. At skin closure or when counted items are no longer used on the sterile field
6. Whenever permanent relief staff enter the case (e.g., during a shift or other personnel change in either the scrub or circulator role)

Instruments, sharps, and miscellaneous items are counted at the same time, according to facility policy.

Procedure for the Count

Items are counted in a specific order:

1. Items on the immediate sterile field (i.e., those on or in the patient)
2. Items on the Mayo stand
3. Items on the back table
4. Items that have been discarded or dropped from the field

The count is performed in a systematic manner. Items should be counted according to their type. For example, count all laparotomy sponges, and then count all 4 × 4 sponges; continue to count all other types of sponges on the field according to their type.

Count suture needles, blades, other small items, and instruments (and their loose parts) as separate groups. The items being counted should be grouped together and accessible for the initial count.

The count is performed audibly, with the circulator and the scrub person participating equally. Both people participating in the count must see the items as they are counted. The circulator and scrub person are required to sign the count on the patient's operative record. This is a legal document that attests to the outcome of the count. Anyone who performs a count, including relief personnel, must sign off their count.

The standard procedure for the count is shown in Box 4.1.

Counting Systems

The most commonly retained item is the surgical sponge. Systems used to collect (confine) and count sponges prevent errors. These include multipocket bags that can be suspended from an IV stand. Counts may be recorded during surgery using a whiteboard. Electronic technology currently in use for the count include bar coding and radiofrequency tagging, in which a chip is embedded in each sponge and can be tracked using a tracking device. These devices are rapidly gaining the approval of professional organizations and may become mandatory in future.

Emergencies and Counts

There may be extreme emergency cases in which the life of the patient is immediately endangered and a count is waived. The

---

BOX 4.1 Standard Procedure for the Surgical Count

What
- Soft goods (textiles) including radiopaque sponges of all types, surgical towels, and packing material (e.g., material used in the nasal cavity to absorb blood)
- Individual suture packages
- Sharps, including intact knife blades, hypodermic needles, suture needles, trocars, and fragments, if broken
- Instruments
- Miscellaneous items such as electrosurgery tips, cranial (Raney type) clips and their cartridges, umbilical and vessel loops, electrosurgery cleaning pads, small bottles and their caps, medical device parts, and any other object that can be lost in the surgical wound

When
- Before the procedure (to establish a baseline)
- Whenever additional items are introduced to the sterile field intraoperatively
- At the start of wound closure
- Before closing any hollow organ
- Before closing a body cavity
- During closure of skin or other final tissue layer
- Whenever permanent relief personnel join the surgical team
- At the request of the surgeon or any other team member

How
- According to the healthcare institution's policy
- In a systematic, deliberate way, without distraction or interruption
- Without deviation from policy and protocol
- In an established sequence by the type of item being counted (e.g., instruments, sponges, sharps)
- By separating or pointing to each and every item and counting them individually
- Audibly and visually; both people performing the count do so aloud, as they see the items being counted

Who
- As designated by healthcare facility policy
- The circulator and scrubbed technologist or nurse
- Other members of the sterile team and circulator

Documentation
- As soon as a count is taken, it is documented on a count sheet and/or whiteboard.
- Whenever new counted items are added to the sterile field, they are immediately entered on the count sheet and/or whiteboard.
- All scrub and circulating personnel are required to sign off the count, validating the numbers and who participated in the counts during surgery.

From Fuller JK: *Surgical technology: Principles and practice*, ed 7, St Louis, 2018, Elsevier.

---

amount of time between the announcement of an incoming emergency and the arrival of the patient in the operating room may be less than 10 minutes. In these few minutes, the surgical team must prepare the operating room, open the case, perform hand antisepsis, and receive the patient. If an initial count is waived, documentation must reflect this and state the rationale. During the case, counts are performed as usual, as the situation permits. Imaging may be performed at the conclusion of the case to demonstrate that no item was seen. Each facility is responsible for publishing protocols and policies regarding waived counts.

Documentation

All counts are documented in the patient record. The documentation includes the names of the individuals who participated in the counts (including relief staff) and their signatures attesting to a correct or incorrect count. Count sheets on which real-time counts are documented may become part of the permanent record, according to facility policy.

A retained item is reported as a sentinel event even if the item is eventually located and the count validated. This requires documentation on an incident report or by other facility protocol. If the item is found, it is documented as a near miss. The report must include the steps taken to find the missing item.

LOST AND RETAINED ITEMS

Loss of sponges, needles, instruments, or other surgical equipment extends anesthesia time, increases patient risk, raises costs, and increases stress on the surgical team. If a surgical sponge or other item is left behind in the patient, it may be spotted on X-ray. However, the extended anesthesia time required for X-ray to be called and an image made available can add risk and expense.

How Items are Lost

The most-recent studies on retained surgical items show that specific scenarios in surgery are more likely to lead to incorrect counts and discrepancies:

- The procedure lasts for more than 8 hours.
- There is multiple staff turnover during a procedure.
- A sponge is used inappropriately (i.e., outside of the usual protocol). For example, a Raytec (4 × 4) sponge is not mounted on a clamp for use in a body cavity.
- There is failure to document items added to the field during surgery.
- The team has not kept track of sponges as they are used.
- The surgical field is cluttered or disorganized.
- The sponge count is performed improperly.

Excessive noise from music, equipment, talking, and cell phones may make it difficult to hear the count.

The scrub must be accountable for sponges as they are used. This requires focused attention to the operative site and concentration on what items are in use. Sponges (and instruments) can easily become "lost" in the body cavity of a deep-bodied or obese patient. Sponges are often found in the folds of drapes, under basins, among the skin prep sponges, or on the floor under the operating table. Small needles are lost when they snag on drapes or other linen and spring off the field. Small items, such as instrument parts, can easily drop into the wound.

How to Search for a Lost Item

If the count is incorrect, the surgeon is notified and the count is repeated. If the count is still incorrect, a search is initiated. Non-sterile team members search non-sterile areas, while scrubbed team members search the wound and sterile field. Normally, the surgical technologist is responsible for searching the back table, Mayo, and any other instrument tables. All trash and waste receptacles are emptied onto an impervious drape, and each piece is searched. As each bag is searched, the contents are rebagged systematically. Equipment on the back table must be shifted to allow a search under instrument trays and basins. The floor around the operating table is thoroughly examined, and team members are asked to step slightly away from the field, because sponges are often found between the team member and the table or patient. A rolling magnet is used to search all floor spaces for metal items. Team members must show the soles of their shoes for inspection, another place where lost needles can be found. The smallest microsurgical needles cannot be seen on X-rays and may be very difficult to spot on or around the surgical field.

If a sponge or needle is not found, an X-ray is usually ordered. If the item is lost during closure, the procedure may be halted until the X-ray is read. However, not all retained items are easily seen on an X-ray. If a lost item is neither found in the room nor revealed on an X-ray, it may still be retained in the wound. In such a case, all layers of the surgical wound may be reopened and searched. If the surgeon is confident that the item has not been left in the wound and the risk of extended anesthesia does not outweigh the risk of a retained object, the X-ray may be ordered in the PACU.

Preventing Retained Items

The problem of retained items and the health consequences are of such significance that safety and professional organizations have instituted conferences, new research studies, and awareness campaigns to try to decrease their incidence. Among the most important messages to operating room teams are the following summary guidelines on preventing retained items, which are derived from both the Association of Surgical Technologists and AORN recommended practices:

- During the count, unnecessary activity and distraction should be curtailed to allow the scrub and RN circulator to focus on the task at hand.
- Standardized procedure should be used during all counts.
- Sharps must be contained within a specific area of the sterile field in a containment device.
- Radiopaque soft goods (e.g., sponges, towels, textiles) should be accounted for during all procedures in which soft goods are used.
- If the surgical sponge pack is banded, the band should be broken and discarded before the count.
- Items are counted as they are added to a case.
- Radiopaque sponges must not be used as wound dressings or in the patient prep.
- All counted items should stay in the operating room or procedure room until the close of surgery.
- The final count is not complete until all sponges used in closing the wound are accounted for.
- Sponges or other counted items dropped on the floor should be retrieved by the circulator and the item shown to the scrub.
- Sponges and other radiopaque items must not be cut for use in the wound.
- Small instrument components such as wing nuts, screws, and pins are counted separately.
- Broken instrument parts are isolated from the setup and accounted for.

- Trash and linen bags must remain in the operating room until the patient has left the room.

Surgical Count and Lost and Retained Items sections from Fuller JK: *Surgical technology: Principles and practice,* ed 7, St Louis, 2018, Elsevier.

CONCLUSION

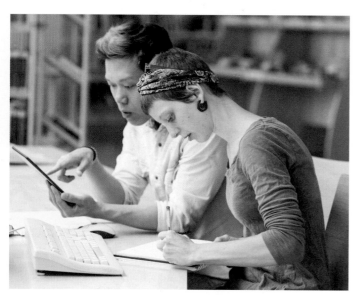

(Copyright © SilviaJansen/iStock/Getty Images.)

Congratulations on completing this review of surgical case management. If you feel ready, complete the chapter review questions and check your answers on the Evolve Resources site. If you feel that you need more review, make your way through the chapter again, focusing on any weak areas.

REVIEW QUESTIONS

1. Handwashing is:
   a. An example of clean surgical technique
   b. An important event-related preventive measure for reducing the incidence of infection
   c. Not a good preventive measure
   d. Surgically clean and a time-related event
2. Which of these practices is **not** safe?
   a. Using an opened sterile bottle for the next case
   b. Standing next to surgeon when passing off a towel for draping
   c. Keeping nonsterile persons 12 inches from the sterile field
   d. Controlling the noise level in the operating room
3. Which of these modes of transmission is **not** common in the hospital setting?
   a. Contaminated food
   b. Dirty hands
   c. Sneezing
   d. Air
4. Which of these is **not** one of the four principles of asepsis?
   a. Handwashing
   b. Aseptic technique with a sterile field
   c. Clean equipment
   d. Clean water
5. Which of these signs are indicative of inflammation?
1. Swelling

2. Pain
3. Loss of function
4. Increased temperature
5. Pus formation
   a. 1, 3, 4
   b. 1, 2, 3, 4
   c. 1, 2, 4, 5
   d. 1, 2, 3, 4, 5
6. What is the difference between the terms *clean* and *sterile*?
   a. *Clean* means that the number of spore-bearing bacteria has been reduced.
   b. *Sterile* means that spore-bearing bacteria have been eliminated.
   c. There is no diffence between the terms.
   d. *Clean* means that fungi have been eliminated.
7. Soaking of a solution through sterile drapes is called:
   a. Contamination
   b. Cross-contamination
   c. Strike-through
   d. Partial contamination
8. What is the center of the sterile field during surgery?
   a. Gowned surgical technologist
   b. Sterile instruments
   c. Draped patient
   d. Gowned surgeon

9. For the table to be considered sterile, the surgical technologist should drape it:
   a. 2 inches from the lower edge of the drape
   b. Only at table height
   c. Only in the center
   d. 2 inches below the top

10. An operating room nurse wants a surgical tech to set up the scheduled noon case at 10 a.m. The tech disagrees with the request, stating that this will increase the risk of contamination. It is not recommended that supplies be left open before a case:
    a. Without the patient's being informed of the length of time that the room has been open
    b. For more than 3 hours
    c. For more than 2 hours
    d. Unless signs have been posted on the doors and the doors have been taped to prevent entry into the room

11. A surgeon wants a medical student who has scrubbed to stand to his left to assist in retraction. The student must pass other sterile personnel;
    a. Right side to right side
    b. Front to front or back to back
    c. Right side to left side
    d. Left side to left side

12. A sterile gown is considered sterile, regardless of the height of the surgical team members who are scrubbed for the case:
    a. In the front, from midchest to tabletop
    b. Until they get blood or bodily fluids on them
    c. On the entire front
    d. All over

13. Which statement about masks is correct?
    a. One must remove and dispose of a mask immediately after leaving any restricted or semirestricted area.
    b. One must wear a mask at all times.
    c. One must remove and dispose of a mask immediately after leaving any restricted, semirestricted, or nonrestricted area.
    d. One must remove and dispose of a mask immediately after leaving any restricted area.

14. Joni is scheduled for breast augmentation. When she arrives at the hospital, a nurse notices that she is wearing a necklace and asks her to remove it. The recommended practice is to:
    a. Keep jewelry covered
    b. Remove all jewelry
    c. Only wear earrings and necklaces
    d. Only wear clean jewelry

15. Aseptic technique is also known as:
    a. Surgically clean technique
    b. Handwashing technique
    c. Scrubbing technique
    d. Sterile technique

16. Coronary artery bypass grafting (CABG) is categorized as wound class:
    a. I
    b. II
    c. III
    d. IV

17. Which four agents are the most likely to be used by terrorists for mass transmission resulting in mortality, panic, and social disruption that could threaten national and world security?
    a. Anthrax, tuberculosis, *Clostridium difficile*, tularemia
    b. Smallpox, monkeypox, avian influenza, anthrax
    c. Anthrax, H1N1 influenza, botulism, smallpox
    d. Smallpox, plague, botulism, tularemia

18. What microorganism is responsible for most SSIs (surgical site infections)?
    a. *Staphylococcus aureus*
    b. *Streptococcus pyogenes*
    c. *Enterococcus faecalis*
    d. *Staphylococcus epidermidis*

19. Which of these diseases is a form of transmissible spongiform encephalopathy caused by prions?
    a. Toxic shock
    b. Creutzfeldt-Jakob disease
    c. Meningitis
    d. Neuritis

20. Cidex is one trade name given to:
    a. Glutaraldehyde
    b. Ethylene oxide
    c. Peracetic acid
    d. Hydrogen peroxide gas plasma

21. What microorganism is an anaerobic gram-positive bacterium responsible for gas gangrene, cellulitis, and fasciitis?
    a. *Helicobacter pylori*
    b. *Staphylococcus aureus*
    c. Prion
    d. *Clostridium perfringens*

22. What microorganism is an aerobic, gram-negative bacillus known to cause gastric ulcers?.
    a. *Clostridium perfringens*
    b. *Staphylococcus aureus*
    c. *Helicobacter pylori*
    d. *Escherichia coli*

23. In which intention of healing does a wound gradually fill in with granulation rather than being sutured?
    a. First
    b. Second
    c. Third
    d. Fourth

24. The first intention wound healing that begins within minutes of an intentional or unintentional injury is known as:
    a. Proliferation
    b. Maturation
    c. Granulation
    d. Inflammatory phase

25. Studies have shown that primary union wound healing occurs from:
    a. End to end
    b. Side to side
    c. Top to bottom
    d. Bottom to top

Surgical Pharmacology

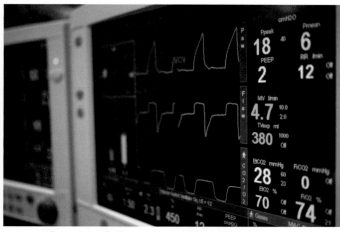

(Copyright © Fivepointsix/iStock/Getty Images.)

Pharmacology—with its great number and variety of drugs and their potential for interaction—poses one of the biggest challenges for most surgical technology students.

What's the best way to learn and remember pharmacology? The best method we have found is simple repetition paired with putting yourself in the patient's shoes. If you've had surgery, recall your experiences, and if you haven't, just imagine the experience.

As you know, there are three phases in surgical case management:

- Preoperative
- Intraoperative
- Postoperative

There are also four phases of general anesthesia, during which specific tasks are performed and certain medications are administered (Table 5.1).

Let's track a patient through a surgery, examining the medications that may be administered, depending on the purpose of the surgery.

PREOPERATIVE DRUGS

These drugs are administered in the holding area to prepare the patient physically and psychologically for surgery.

Hydration

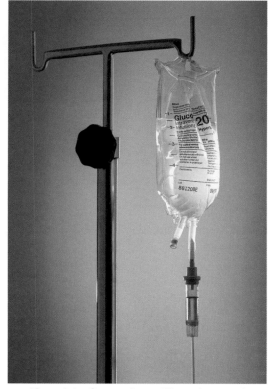

(Copyright © moodboard/Getty Images.)

TABLE 5.1	Phases of Anesthesia
Anesthesia Phase	**What's Going On**
Phase 1: preinduction	Placement of noninvasive monitoring devices on the patient Preparation of suction, EKG leads, and IV line by anesthesia care provider (ACP)
Phase 2: induction	Administration of induction agent Descent of patient through the five stages of anesthesia: **Stage 1: analgesia** • Begins with administration of anesthetic agent • Ends when patient loses consciousness • Amplified hearing at the end of this stage • Amnesia **Stage 2: excitement** • Quiet environment required (hearing is the last faculty lost by the patient in anesthesia) • Tensed muscles • Swallowing reflexes (and sometimes laryngospasm) • Vomiting reflexes • Irregular breathing or breath-holding • Delirium • Pupil dilation • Tachycardia • Hypertension **Stage 3: surgical anesthesia** • Depression of vital functions • Pupil constriction • Regular respiration • Absence of movement (loss or temporary depression of muscle reflexes) • Assessment of adequacy of anesthesia depth by anesthesia provider **Stage 4: overdose** • Respiratory arrest • Vasomotor collapse • Widely dilated pupils • Relaxed muscles
Phase III (maintenance)	Continued maintenance of unconsciousness, using a variety of anesthetic agents, by the anesthesiologist (balanced anesthesia): • IV • Gaseous • Vapor
Phase IV (emergence)	Reduction of all anesthetics Preparation of patient for return to consciousness Administration of reversal agent
Phase 5: recovery	Placement of patient on stretcher Transport of patient to PACU to regain consciousness Continuous monitoring of vital signs

A patient may be given any of several intravenous (IV) solutions to help ensure homeostasis and safe anesthesia, depending on the patient and the surgery.

0.9% Sodium Chloride (NaCl) (Isotonic)

This is a salt solution.
- Agent of choice for fluid replacement or simple hydration
- Used for the transfusion of blood products because it does not induce hemolysis (destruction) of blood cells

Dextrose (D)

Dextrose is a sugar solution.
- Used to hydrate the surgical patient, spare body protein (by providing a source of energy), and enhance liver function.
- Used for the temporary treatment of circulatory insufficiency and shock due to hypovolemia in the absence of plasma extender
- Also used for early treatment, with plasma, of fluid loss due to burns
- *Not* used in the transfusion of blood products; causes hemolysis of blood cells

Lactated Ringer's Solution (LR)

This salt solution is also referred to as Ringer lactate (RL).
- Replenishes the patient's electrolytes
- Used for rehydration to stimulate renal activity
- Also used to replace fluid lost from burns or severe diarrhea
- Not advised for patients with liver disease, Addison disease, severe pH imbalance, shock or cardiac failure

Ionosol B

This solution is also known as MB&T.
- Used for maintenance and replacement of electrolytes
- Provides water, electrolytes, and carbohydrates to cover hydration, insensible water loss, and urine production

PlasmaLyte or Isolyte E

These solutions are used to treat massive loss of water and electrolytes.
- Often used in the setting of uncontrolled vomiting or diarrhea, shock, burns, or multiple blood transfusions

Physical and Psychological Preparation for Surgery
Sedatives

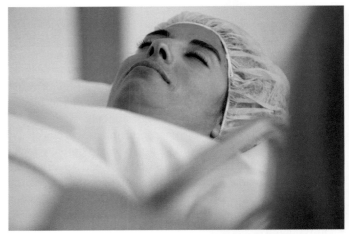

(Copyright © Wavebreakmedia Ltd./Wavebreak Media/Getty Images.)

These medications relieve anxiety; some produce mild drowsiness and may have amnestic and antiemetic effects. The main adverse effect is respiratory depression.

Benzodiazepines. At low dosages, these drugs exert an anxiolytic effect (relief of anxiety); at higher doses they induce sedation and anterograde amnesia.

- Diazepam (Valium)
- Lorazepam (Midazolam)
- Midazolam (Versed) (most commonly used)

Gastric Agents

Nil per os (nothing by mouth; NPO) status is instituted for a patient undergoing elective surgery, but there will still be acidic gastric secretions in the stomach that may be aspirated if the patient vomits during the induction of anesthesia. This could in turn result in the development of a condition known as aspiration pneumonitis.

A patient who must undergo emergency surgery is at even greater risk because there has been no fasting to empty the stomach, increasing the likelihood of vomiting of food or secretions and therefore increasing the risk of aspiration.

Certain conditions put patients at even higher risk for aspiration, even when NPO status is instituted:

- Gastrointestinal obstruction
- History of gastrointestinal reflux disease
- Diabetes
- Obesity
- Labor
- Scheduled cesarean section

Gastric agents commonly used in surgery. These medications are generally used to control stomach acid.

- Antacids
  - Sodium citrate with citric acid (Bicitra): This drug given before surgery to neutralize the acidity of stomach contents by causing them to be metabolized to sodium bicarbonate.
- H_2-receptor antagonists
  - Cimetidine (Tagamet)
  - Famotidine (Pepcid)
  - Ranitidine (Zantac)
- Proton pump inhibitors
  - Protonix IV (reduces gastric acid in 20 minutes)
- Antiemetic and gastrointestinal prokinetics.
  - These agents are administered before surgery to reduce nausea and minimize the possibility of postoperative nausea and vomiting (PONV) in at-risk patients:
    - Preadolescents
    - Obese people
    - People with diabetes
    - People with a history of gastroesophageal reflux disease
    - Women in labor or undergoing scheduled cesarean section
    - Patients receiving opioids, barbiturates, or etomidate
    - Patients with gastrointestinal obstruction
  - Antiemetic drugs include:
    - Metoclopramide (Reglan)
    - Droperidol (Inapsine)
    - Ondansetron (Zofran)

Analgesics

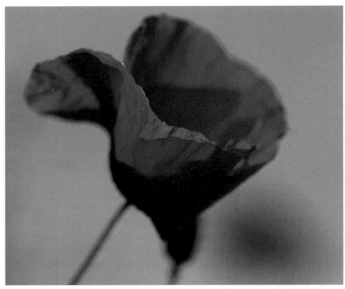

(Copyright © Andriy Solovyov/Hemera/Getty Images.)

Pain relievers are often given before surgery to trauma patients and to patients who will require the insertion of invasive monitors before surgery. The most commonly administered analgesic agents are opioids (narcotics)—morphine, heroin, and other drugs derived from the opium poppy (shown here), as well as synthetic versions of these drugs.

Commonly administered analgesics

- Morphine (natural opioid)
- Meperidine (Demerol; synthetic opioid)
- Fentanyl (Sublimaze; synthetic opioid)

Facts to remember

- These agents induce analgesia and mild sedation; this helps the anesthesiologist reduce the amount of anesthesia needed for the surgical procedure.
- **Nausea and vomiting** is sometimes seen with these agents.
- **Slowed respiration and intestinal motility** is expected with these drugs. (When there is slowed respiration, it is monitored with a **pulse oximeter**).
- Opioids are **contraindicated** in patients undergoing ambulatory surgery because of the prohibitively intensive monitoring they require.

Anticholinergics

These agents block the action of neurotransmitter acetylcholine, inhibiting the transmission of **parasympathetic nerve** impulses.

- Not routinely used but are indicated in specific instances to inhibit mucous secretions in the respiratory and digestive tract (**antisialagogue effect**)
- Commonly used anticholinergics:
  - Atropine
  - Glycopyrrolate (potent antisialagogue effect)
  - Scopolamine (three times as potent as antisialagogue effect)
- Preferred for these procedures:

- During **induction** (endotracheal tube insertion)
- Bronchoscopy
- Maxillofacial surgery

Antibiotics

These drugs, also known as **antimicrobial agents**, are used to prevent and to treat infections caused by pathogenic (disease-causing) microorganisms. There are six major groups of antibiotics that every student should remember, each with a different means of combating microorganisms (Fig. 5.1):

Aminoglycosides. This class of antibiotics is derived from various strains of the *Actinomyces* bacteria genus.

- **Interfere with protein synthesis** by binding to bacterial ribosomes, meaning that there are bactericidal and narrow spectra of action
- Active only against **aerobic gram-negative bacteria and some methicillin-resistant strains**
- Major adverse effects: nephrotoxicity and ototoxicity
- Usually administered **IV** but given orally during colorectal surgery to reduce bacterial load in the bowel
- Commonly administered aminoglycosides
  - Amikacin (Amikin)
  - Gentamicin (Garamycin)
  - Kanamycin (Kantrex)
  - Tobramycin (Nebcin)
  - Neomycin (Neobiotic)
  - Streptomycin

Cephalosporins. These broad-spectrum antibiotics have a wide range of uses.

- Derived from bacteria in the *Acremonium* species
- Bactericidal, blocking an enzyme needed to strengthen the bacteria cell wall and causing cell lysis (rupture)
- Various generations of cephalosporins are active against many different microbes, depending on their mutagenic characteristics:
- **First-generation cephalosporins** are active against many gram-positive and some gram-negative microbes:
  - Cefazolin (Ancef, Kefzol)
  - Cefadroxil (Duricef, Ultracef)
  - Cefapirin (Cefadryl)
  - Cephalexin (Keflex, Keflet)
  - Cephalothin (Keflin)
  - Cefradine (Anspor, Velosef)
- **Second-generation drugs** are effective against a wider variety of gram-negative microbes but work against fewer gram-positive ones:
  - Cefoxitin (Mefoxin)
  - Cefprozil (Cefzil)
  - Cefaclor (Ceclor, Keflor, Raniclor)
  - Cefmetazole (Zefazone)
  - Cefotetan (Cefotan)
  - Cefuroxime (Ceftin, Zinacef, Zinnat)
- **Third-generation agents** are effective against wider range of gram-negative microbes than second-generation drugs are but are less effective against gram-positive microbes. Sometimes they are used in hospital-acquired infections.
- Cefotaxime (Claforan)

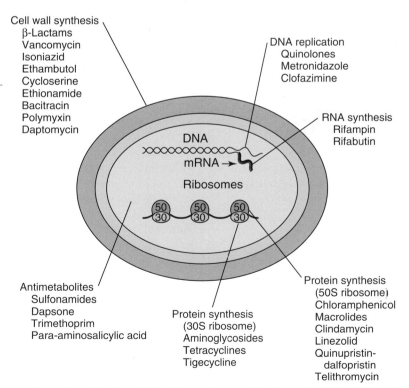

FIG. 5.1 Basic sites of antibiotic activity. (From Murray PR, Rosenthal KS, Pfaller MA: Medical microbiology, ed 8, Philadelphia, 2016, Elsevier.)

- Cefixime (Suprax)
- Cefoperazone (Cefobid)
- Ceftazidime (Fortum, Fortaz)
- Ceftizoxime (Cefizox)
- Ceftriaxone (Rocephin)
- **Fourth-generation medications** are effective against a wider range of gram-positive and gram-negative microbes, including meningitis bugs and *Pseudomonas aeruginosa*:
  - Cefepime (Cepimax, Maxcef, Maxipime)
- **Fifth-generation antibiotics** have been reported to have powerful antipseudomonal properties and to exert potent effects against methicillin-resistant *Staphylococcus aureus* (MRSA).
  - Ceftobiprole (Zeftera, Zevtera)

Penicillins

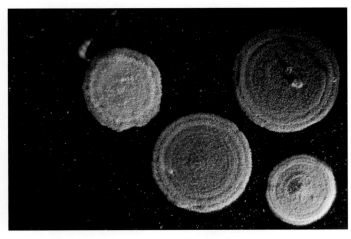

(Copyright © Eugeny Korshenkov/Hemera/Getty Images.)

Penicillin, discovered in 1928, was the **first true antibiotic**. It and its relatives are used as prophylaxis against infection of surgical sites.

- Prescribed before dental or other medical procedures to prevent bacterial infection of the heart (**endocarditis**) in patients with prosthetic heart valves
- Derived from *Penicillium* species molds (see image).
- **Bactericidal**; acts by blocking an enzyme that strengthens the bacterial cell wall, resulting in the eventual rupture of the cell
- Cross-reactivity among penicillin and some of the cephalosporin antibiotics
- Some bacterial resistance involving the production of **penicillinase**, an enzyme that breaks down the drug molecule, inactivating it.
- Types of penicillin drugs
  - **Natural penicillins** are inexpensive and are associated with low toxicity.
    - Penicillin G
    - Penicillin V
    - Penicillin benzathine G

- **Aminopenicillins** are chemically altered by the addition of an amino group that makes them more effective against gram-negative species.
  - Ampicillin
  - Amoxicillin
  - Bacampicillin
- **Penicillinase-resistant penicillins** are semisynthetic. They are effective against strains of bacteria that produce penicillinase, but some microbes develop resistance to these drugs. MRSA is resistant to this drug group.
  - Flucloxacillin
  - Cloxacillin
  - Dicloxacillin
  - Nafcillin
  - Oxacillin
- **Broad-spectrum penicillins** are semisynthetics, chemically altered to render them effective against gram-negative microbes.
  - Mezlocillin
  - Piperacillin
  - Ticarcillin

Tetracyclines. These drugs were the first broad-spectrum antibiotics.
- Derived from cultures of *Streptomyces* species bacteria
- Binds to the bacterial ribosomal subunit, interfering with protein synthesis
- Never administered to pediatric patients, because they permanently stain the teeth yellow.
- Commonly prescribed tetracycline drugs
  - Tetracycline hydrochloride
  - Minocycline
  - Oxytetracycline (Terramycin)
  - Doxycycline

Macrolides. These antibiotics are derived from isolates of *Streptomyces erythreus*.
- **Inhibits bacterial protein synthesis** by binding to the prokaryotic ribosomal subunit and penetrating the cell walls of the gram-positive organism; bactericidal against several gram-positive bacteria (e.g., *Legionella*)
- May cause diarrhea, nausea, and vomiting
- Commonly prescribed macrolide drugs
  - Erythromycin
  - Azithromycin
  - Clarithromycin

Miscellaneous Antibiotics

- Clindamycin is given when a patient is allergic to sulfa or penicillin antibiotics.
- Metronidazole (Flagyl) is used for systemic prophylaxis in elective surgery of the colon and rectum.
- Vancomycin is given when a patient is allergic to sulfa or penicillin drugs. The decision to administer it depends on the likely pathogen, which is deduced from local epidemiology and susceptibility patterns, as well as the potentially catastrophic nature of an infection. Vancomycin is often combined with drugs in the cephalosporin group.

INTRAOPERATIVE DRUGS

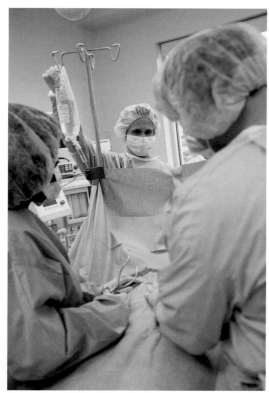

(Copyright © Jupiterimages/Photos.com/Getty Images.)

Generally, the medications administered intraoperatively are the same ones given before surgery:

- IV fluids
- Antibiotics
- Muscle relaxants
- Balanced anesthesia, in which the anesthesiologist alters the ratio of three types of anesthetic agents to one another on the basis of the duration of surgery and how the patient responds.
  - **Inhalation agents** (e.g., isoflurane, desflurane, sevoflurane)
  - **Gaseous agents** (e.g., nitrous oxide)
  - **IV anesthetic agents** (e.g., propofol)

Anesthesia for Same-Day Surgery

Patients undergoing same-day (ambulatory) surgery receive one of two types of anesthesia:

Local Anesthesia

This type of anesthesia is used for minor procedures. Generally it consists of:

- **Lidocaine**, a fast-acting anesthetic agent, combined with epinephrine, a vasoconstrictor, in a 1:100,000 or 1:200,000 dilution; the epinephrine helps the anesthetic agent last longer and minimizes blood loss.
- **Marcaine**, a slow-acting anesthetic agent, combined with epinephrine, a vasoconstrictor, in a 1:100,000 or 1:200,000 dilution; the epinephrine helps the anesthetic agent last longer and minimizes blood loss.
- **Lidocaine and marcaine** may be mixed together in a 1:1 ratio.

Regional Anesthesia

Various types of regional (versus general) anesthesia are used, depending on the area in which surgery is to be performed. Anesthesia of a single nerve or group of nerves or total spinal cord block is possible. Commonly used types of regional anesthesia include:

- The **Bier block** is used in limb surgeries in which nerve block is possible for short durations.
- **Epidural and caudal blocks** are used in cesarean sections, urologic surgery, and rectal surgery. Local anesthetic is injected into the epidural space of the spinal cord.
- The **spinal block** is used in orthopedic, genitourinary, and gynecologic cases when general anesthesia poses a significant physiological risk to the patient. A local anesthetic is injected into the subarachnoid space of the spinal cord.

POSTOPERATIVE DRUGS

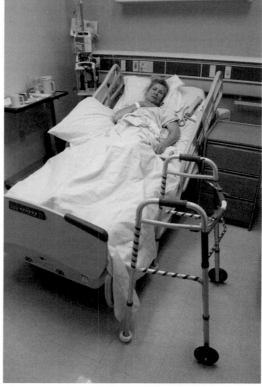

(Copyright © Ken Hurst/Hemera/Getty Images.)

These agents are given to keep the patient comfortable and hasten recovery.

- **IV fluids** are continued to help maintained homeostasis and help the body excrete anesthesia drugs by way of the urinary tract. Having an IV drip in place also makes the administration of some medications easier.
- **Analgesic drugs** are provided as needed to control pain if the patient is admitted to the hospital for a few days. Often a patient-controlled analgesia (PCA) pump will be provided to help the patient control pain as required with the use of a drug such as morphine.
- Intravenous **antibiotics** are given if the patient is admitted to the hospital; patients who undergo same-day surgery will

be prescribed oral antibiotics prophylactically by the surgeon after the procedure.

CONCLUSION

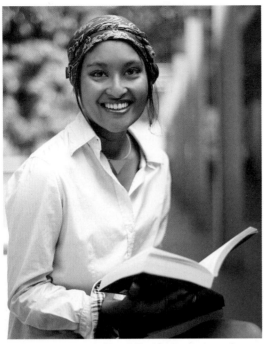

(Copyright © Tassii/E+/Getty Images.)

Congratulations! You've completed this review of surgical pharmacology. If you feel ready, complete the chapter review questions and check your answers on the Evolve Resources site; if you need a little more review, make your way through the chapter again.

▮ REVIEW QUESTIONS

1. This device is placed on a highly vascular area of the body (digit or ear lobe), making continuous readings oxygen saturation readings available.
   a. Thermometer
   b. Pulse oximeter
   c. Vascular monitor
   d. Blood pressure cuff

2. During general anethesia, certain drugs are used to achieve paralysis of all muscles. What device is used to secure and maintain 100% oxygen saturation?
   a. Mechanical ventilator
   b. Perfusion machine
   c. Oxygen saturation monitor
   d. Bag-valve mask

3. Monitored anesthesia care (MAC) is continuous patient monitoring provided during regional anesthesia. During this time, an ACP (anesthesia care provider) admini sters:
   a. Sedative and anxiolytic drugs as needed
   b. Sedative and antidepressant drugs as needed
   c. Sedatives and blood transfusions as needed
   d. Sedative and antipsychotic drugs as needed

4. Malignant hyperthermia is a rare physiological response to volatile anesthetic agents and succinylcholine. It can be reversed with the administration of:
   a. Benzodiazepines
   b. Narcotics
   c. Sevoflurane
   d. Dantrolene

5. The state of balance in physiological function is known as:
   a. Homeostasis
   b. Hemostasis
   c. Hemotocrit
   d. Hemodialysis

6. Fentanyl is a:
   a. Neuromuscular blocking agent
   b. Benzodiazepine
   c. Sedative/hypnotic
   d. Narcotic

7. Propofol is a:
   a. Neuromuscular blocking agent
   b. Benzodiazepine
   c. Sedative/hypnotic
   d. Narcotic

8. Diazepam is a:
   a. Neuromuscular blocking agent
   b. Benzodiazepine
   c. Sedative/hypnotic
   d. Narcotic

9. Succinylcholine, used to paralyze skeletal muscles, is a:
   a. Neuromuscular blocking agent
   b. Benzodiazepine
   c. Sedative/hypnotic
   d. Narcotic

10. This agent is a colorless, odorless, and tasteless gas with mild analgesic and amnestic properties:
    a. Sevoflurane
    b. Nitrogen gas
    c. Nitrous oxide
    d. Oxygen gas

11. _____ is the agent of choice for fluid replacement or simple hydration and, because it does not cause hemolysis of blood cells, when blood products are being transfused.
    a. 0.9% Sodium chloride (NaCl)
    b. Dextrose
    c. Inosol B
    d. Ringer lactate

12. All of the following drugs belong to the benzodiazepine family **except**:
    a. Diazepam (Valium)
    b. Lorazepam (Ativan)
    c. Midazolam (Versed)
    d. Pantoprazole (Protonix)

13. Which agent is administered before surgery to reduce nausea and minimize the possibility of postoperative nausea and vomiting in at-risk patients?
    a. Metoclopramide (Reglan)
    b. Diazepam (Valium)
    c. Ringer Lactate
    d. Pantoprazole (Protonix)

14. A 68-year-old patient is scheduled for hip nailing. The patient's history indicates that he is a longtime smoker. The anesthesia care provider wants to instill of a local anesthetic into the subarachnoid space for better postoperative recovery. This is called:
    a. Spinal anesthesia
    b. Epidural anesthesia
    c. Perfusion block
    d. Stellate ganglion block

15. _____ and _____promote rapid induction and recovery and offer the fastest onset of induction, emergence, and recovery.
    a. Nitrous oxide and oxygen
    b. Halothane and desflurane
    c. Desflurane and sevoflurane
    d. Nitrous oxide and halothane

16. The medical record from a patient's previous surgery states that she sustained postoperative nausea and vomiting (PONV). Nitrous oxide and morphine were administered. What drug would an anesthesia care provider administer to prevent this problem in future surgeries?
    a. Metoclopramide (Reglan)
    b. Diazepam (Valium)
    c. Pantoprazole (Protonix)
    d. Ringer lactate

17. Ketamine, a short-acting induction and IV or IM maintenance agent, helps maintain the patient's airway. It is safe for use in small children and burn patients. When administered in large doses, however, it may cause:
    a. Respiratory depression
    b. Hallucinations
    c. Hallucinations and respiratory depression
    d. Thrombocytopenia

18. The surgical technologist in the circulator role (STCR) is often asked by the anesthesia care provider (ACP) to apply cricoid pressure to:
    a. Help the ACP visualize the vocal cords
    b. Prevent regurgitation of stomach contents
    c. Prevent salivation
    d. Prevent regurgitation of stomach contents and help the ACP visualize the vocal cords

19. All of these drugs belong to the cephalosporin family **except**:
    a. Ancef,
    b. Kefzol
    c. Keflex
    d. Kanamycin

20. A 5-year-old scheduled for dental restoration is noted to have heavy yellow staining of the teeth. The patient's mother mentions that the primary care physician treated the child for bacterial infection 2 years ago. What antibiotic agent should not be given to pediatric patients?
    a. Amoxicillin
    b. Tetracycline
    c. Cephalosporin
    d. Macrolides

21. Fentanyl citrate is the generic name for:
    a. Toradol
    b. Sublimaze
    c. Morphine
    d. Ketamine

22. Before the induction of Bier block anesthesia, the limb in question is Esmarched, after which a double-cuffed tourniquet is inflated around the limb. Esmarching is also known as:
    a. Exsanguination
    b. Evisceration
    c. Embolization
    d. Extravasation

23. Metabolic processing of a drug within the body, including absorption, distribution, biotransformation, and excretion, is known as:
    a. Pharmacodynamics
    b. Pharmacokinetics
    c. Pharmaco-hemodynamics
    d. Homeostasis

24. At this stage, anesthesia is so deep that cardiovascular and respiratory function is compromised to the point of collapse as a result of depression of brain centers.
    a. Stage 1
    b. Stage 2
    c. Stage 3
    d. Stage 4

25. In one phase of anesthesia, the airway is managed with the use of an LMA (larygeal mask airway). Which phase is this?
    a. Preinduction
    b. Induction
    c. Maintenance
    d. Emergence

Professionalism

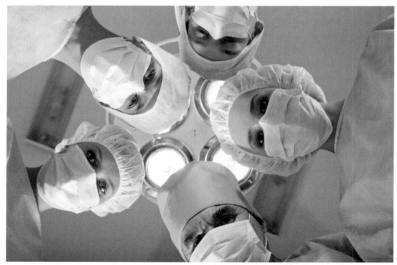

(Copyright © Dmitriy Shironosov/Hemera/Getty Images.)

Just about all of us can recall an encounter with someone working in a professional capacity—a healthcare provider, a college professor—who impressed you with his or her competence, courtesy, and kindness. Most of us, unfortunately, have also dealt with someone who left us feeling uninformed, ignored, or even insulted. As medical professionals, we must make a conscious effort to do our jobs to the best of our ability and inspire confidence in and foster a rapport with our patients.

In this chapter, we'll cover a wide range of topics that you will need to understand not only for your certification examination but also to do your job well and in accordance with the law.

CREDENTIALING

Demonstrating Competence

There are several ways of exhibiting competence in your field:

- *Certification:* Becoming certified in surgical technology by passing a certification examination (i.e., the NBSTSA or NCCT assessment for which you're using this text to study) is a voluntary demonstration of competency and the least restrictive of the three methods discussed here.

- *Registration:* Every state requires surgical technologists to register in that state before practicing.

- *Licensure:* Attaining licensure by fulfilling a state's requirements in regard to education, competence, and practice is the most restrictive of the three means of demonstrating competence.

Professional Organizations

Many different organizations work to ensure safety in healthcare and among the American public. Joining the appropriate groups can help you stay up to date on the most recent developments and reassure patients, family members, and co-workers that you care about doing the best job possible.

- *Association of Surgical Technologists.* The AST, a professional membership organization, is devoted to ensuring that surgical technologists are up to date on the latest skills and techniques.
- *National Board of Surgical Technology and Surgical Assisting.* As you know, the NBSTSA is a certification body for surgical technology and surgical assisting.
- *Council on Surgical and Perioperative Safety.* The CSPS seeks to ensure that patients receive the safest surgical care possible.
- *American College of Surgeons.* The ACS is the main American representative body for surgeons.
- *Association of Perioperative Nurses.* The APN is an organization representing nurses who work in a perioperative role.
- *Centers for Disease Control and Prevention.* This federal agency, better known as the CDC, is a division of the U.S. Department of Health and Human Services (HHS). It is responsible for educating the public on health topics and also monitors and works to prevent and contain disease outbreaks.
- *Food and Drug Administration.* The FDA, another division of the HHS, approves and regulates medical devices and medications.
- *The Joint Commission.* This organization sets standards for health care quality and conducts assessments of participating facilities to ensure compliance.
- *Occupational Safety and Health Administration.* This division of the U.S. Department of Labor, better known as OSHA, monitors and enforces workplace safety.
- *Commission on Accreditation of Allied Health Educational Programs.* The CAAHEP is an accreditation body for educational programs in health care.
- *Accreditation Review Council on Education in Surgical Technology and Surgical Assisting.* ARC-STSA is a committee on accreditation that reports and makes accreditation recommendations to CAAHEP.
- *Accrediting Bureau of Health Education Schools.* The ABHES accredits surgical technology programs; once a program has gained approval, its graduates may sit the CST exam.

COMMUNICATION IN THE WORKPLACE

No matter how good your surgical technology skills, if you are not an effective communicator, you will not be able do your job well.

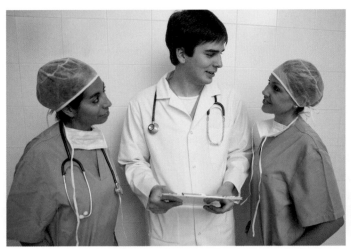

(Copyright © Wavebreakmedia Ltd/Wavebreak Media/Getty Images.)

Effective and Ineffective Communication

Ineffective modes of communication include:

- False reassurance: telling someone that things will be fine when, in fact, they may not
- Defensiveness: reacting angrily when one feels that one is being blamed
- Judgmental behavior: judging others' appearance, clothes, and behaviors
- Inhibition of communication: making it difficult to communicate productively with others

An effective communicator:

- Asks **open-ended questions** (rather than yes-or-no questions) to elicit more information and help the other person express him- or herself
- Engages in **active listening**, giving the speaker his or her full attention
- Asks for **clarification** when something is not clear or it is necessary to ensure that all parties are on the same page
- Is **accepting of input** from others
- Practices **conflict-management skills**: negotiating, bargaining, collaboration
- Engages in **cooperative behaviors** such as open communication
- Knows how to differentiate **message** (any communication containing information) and **meaning** (the intention behind the message [reading between the lines])
- Is able to recognize and interpret **verbal** (spoken) and **nonverbal** (body language, eye contact) communication

Leadership Styles

The surgical technologist who also functions as a leader has several options for managing people in the workplace. Each leadership style has its benefits and drawbacks, and not every style of leading is appropriate in every situation.

- *Autocratic.* There's just one leader, and everyone does things in that person's way.
- *Democratic.* The members of the team work together to make decisions.
- *Laissez-faire.* The leader exerts little or no control, leaving the team members to their own devices.

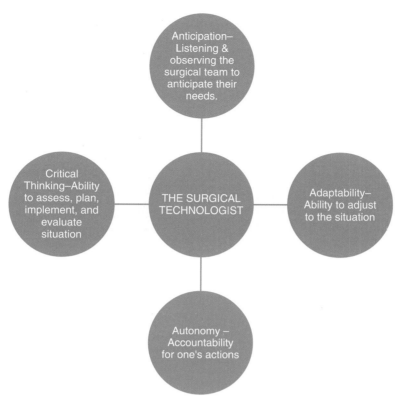

FIG. 6.1 The motto of the AST is *Aeger primo*, Latin for "The patient comes first." Fulfilling this motto requires the surgical technologist to demonstrate attributes.

SURGICAL CONSCIENCE

In addition to solid job skills and the ability to communicate well, professionalism requires the surgical technologist to have what is known as *surgical conscience*. This "conscience" involves:

- Strict adherence to sterile technique
- Accountability, honesty, and integrity in the delivery of quality patient care (including the capacity to speak up if you compromise the sterile field) (Fig. 6.1)
- The understanding that one must advocate for the patient and quality of care, including controlling costs where possible. For instance, it's crucial for the surgical technologist to review the surgeon's preference card before a procedure and refrain from opening supplies that might not be called for during the surgery.

Emotional Development of the Surgical Patient

Always be mindful that a person scheduled for surgery is a member of a special population. Whatever the surgery might be—therapeutic, reconstructive, or cosmetic—the patient will not be the same after surgery. Take, for example, a woman who is to undergo mastectomy. Making the decision to have this surgery is difficult. The surgery and its aftereffects will influence her self-esteem, her sex drive, and how she feels about herself as a woman. It is the obligation of the surgical technologist to treat all surgical patients with compassion and to serve as an advocate on their behalf.

The members of certain populations are more vulnerable and often have special needs as they face surgery:

- Pediatric patients
- Geriatric patients
- Immunocompromised patients
- Diabetic patients
- Pregnant women
- Trauma patients
- Bariatric patients
- Physically or mentally challenged patients
- People who are isolated
- Patients with substance abuse issues

Anyone responsible for advocating for patients or working closely with others must understand what makes people tick, especially in stressful environments such as the operating room.

Pioneering psychologist Abraham Maslow boiled this information down into what has become known as Maslow's Hierarchy of Needs (Fig. 6.2):

- *Physiological.* This includes things needed for survival (e.g., oxygen, water, homeostasis, shelter).
- *Safety.* We seek freedom from danger and poverty.
- *Love and belonging.* Almost everyone desires a feeling of acceptance in social groups.
- *Esteem.* We want to be respected by others and to respect ourselves as well.
- *Self-actualization.* We have the desire or need to achieve our full potential, especially after a life-changing event such as surgery.

Another renowned psychologist, Erik Erikson, formulated with his wife, Joan Erikson, what they called psychosocial stages, in which a person must fulfill tasks of development over his or her lifespan. Success or failure in dealing with these tasks can help explain a person's behavior.

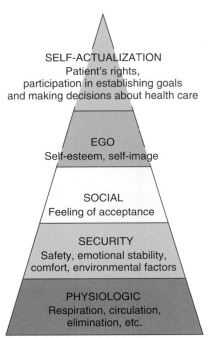

SELF-ACTUALIZATION
Patient's rights,
participation in establishing goals
and making decisions about health care

EGO
Self-esteem, self-image

SOCIAL
Feeling of acceptance

SECURITY
Safety, emotional stability,
comfort, environmental factors

PHYSIOLOGIC
Respiration, circulation,
elimination, etc.

FIG. 6.2 Maslow's hierarchy of needs as related to surgical patient needs during perioperative care. (From Phillips N: Berry & Kohn's operating room technique, ed 13, St Louis, 2017, Elsevier.)

- *Infancy (Birth–1 Year): Trust Versus Mistrust*
  - The infant depends on its mother for nurture, sustenance, and love and ideally begins to experience a sense of trust and hope regarding its place in the world. An infant who is not nurtured and loved and does not develop trust and hope may have trouble learning to trust and love others.
- *Early Childhood (1–3 Years): Autonomy Versus Shame and Doubt*
  - Toddlers begin to develop control over their body functions, as well as some degree of autonomy, and they experience conflict when told no, shamed, embarrassed, or forced to be dependent. A toddler who successfully navigates this stage will emerge with budding willpower and self-control. Failure can result in low self-esteem and too much dependence on others.
- *Preschool (3–6 Years): Initiative Versus Guilt*
  - Children of this age begin to interact with one another—devising games, making plans—in play, at school, and in other contexts and start developing interpersonal skills. Taking the initiative can result in guilt when it is done against the wishes of parents or other authority figures or results in conflict with others. Success in this stage produces a sense of initiative coupled with an understanding of others' rights. Failure can damage self-confidence and stifle initiative and creativity.
- *School-Age (6–12 Years): Industry Versus Inferiority*
  - A school-age child's universe has expanded to include school, sports, and other activities that reward hard work and initiative. Fulfilling goals and achieving success can help the child gain a sense of confidence in his or her abilities; failure can lead the child to develop a persistent belief in his or her inferiority.

- *Adolescence (12–18 Years): Identity Versus Role Confusion*
  - Puberty brings dramatic changes in children's bodies and emotions. The teen years are a time during which the child worries about appearance and tries on various roles and styles in a search for an identity, separate from the parents', that will carry him or her into adulthood. Peer groups take on even greater importance, and the desire to fit in is strong. Success in this stage is marked by the development of a positive adult identity and lifestyle; failure can result in mental illness, an unsettled or even criminal lifestyle, and an inability to settle into adulthood.
- *Young Adulthood (18–30 Years): Intimacy Versus Isolation*
  - If adolescence has gone well, a child enters adulthood with a solid self-identity and a sense of confidence. The struggle in this new stage is the search for a partner: Success brings someone with whom the young adult can share his or her life and lean on in times of trouble; failure results in isolation and loneliness.
- *Adulthood (30–65 Years): Generativity Versus Stagnation*
  - The struggle of adulthood is trying to function as a productive member of society: Success means contributing as a citizen, as an employee, perhaps as a parent, and in other ways as well. Failure is marked by stagnation and a feeling that one is not contributing.
- *Old Age (65 Years and Beyond): Ego Integrity Versus Despair*
  - Old age is a time of reminiscence and reflection. Elders assess their lives and either feel fulfillment on seeing what they've accomplished, as well as a sense of acceptance, or experience despair at having reached the end of their lives without achieving what they wanted.

The Eriksons' theories serve as excellent guidelines for assessment that allow the surgical technologist to anticipate issues in surgical case management and help ensure positive outcomes for patients of all ages.

LEGAL ISSUES

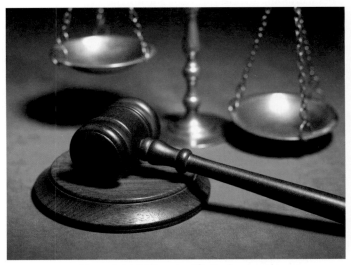

(Copyright © Creatas/Getty Images.)

Working as a medical professional requires **accountability**: not only a degree of legal liability—responsibility under the law for adhering to certain professional standards—but also a duty to patients and co-workers. You'll need to be familiar with certain legal terms and concepts when you take your certification exam.

Criminal Versus Civil

There are two main branches of law: civil and criminal.

- **Criminal law** involves the commission of acts—for instance, theft, assault, or murder—known as **crimes** that violate local, state, or federal statutes.
- Civil law is the resolution of **torts**: wrongful actions, intentional or unintentional.

Torts in Health Care

- A healthcare provider who stops caring for a patient without a good reason and doesn't give the patient the chance to find another provider is committing **abandonment.**
- Spreading false information about another person that results in damage to that person's reputation, ability to earn a living, or both is known as **defamation.** There are two kinds:
  - **Libel** is verbal defamation.
  - **Slander** is any defamatory statement that is published or broadcast.
- Failure to fulfill the accepted standard of care is **neglect.**
- Any intentional act (or omission of action) on the part of a medical professional that is not in keeping with standards of practice, especially one that results in the injury or death of a patient, is considered **malpractice.**
- Injury or illness that is sustained in the healthcare setting or caused by a medical professional is called **iatrogenic injury.** (It's important to remember that not all iatrogenic injuries are considered negligence or malpractice, however—complications of surgery, for example, are classed as iatrogenic because they occur as a result of a medical procedure.)

Box 6.1 shows how torts are categorized as intentional or unintentional. (Some torts, as you might surmise, also qualify as crimes.)

Legal Latin

As you know from your reading of Chapter 1, many words are built on Latin roots. The legal profession, too, draws on Latin for many of its concepts and sayings. Here are a few that you're likely to encounter:

- *Aeger primo*, which means "The patient first," is the motto of the AST.
- *Primum non nocere* means "Above all, do no harm."
- *Res ipsa loquitur* means "The thing speaks for itself." In the healthcare setting, this phrase refers to an act so obviously below the standard of practice that negligence is assumed.
- *Respondeat superior*, meaning "Let the master answer," refers to the fact that in many jurisdictions, your employer is legally responsible for what you do in the course of your employment.

BOX 6.1   Intentional and Unintentional Torts

Tort classification	Description
Intentional	Any willful act that causes harm or distress to another person
Assault	A threat of imminent physical or emotional harm against another person (e.g., intimidating a patient)
Battery	Unwanted physical contact with another person (e.g., a physical attack, touching or treating a patient without consent)
Larceny	Taking something belonging to another person without that person's consent
Defamation	Spreading false information that damages the reputation or livelihood of the subject of the information
False imprisonment	Restraining a person against his or her will (e.g., with physical restraints or the use of drugs)
Infliction of emotional distress	Deliberately causing upset to another person
Invasion of privacy	Violating a person's right to be left alone (e.g., taking photographs or releasing other information without a patient's consent)
Perjury	Lying or falsifying information despite being under oath
Unintentional	Any unintentional act that causes harm or distress to another person

Consent

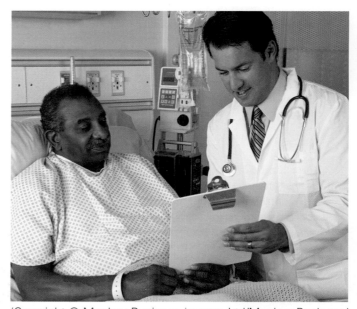

(Copyright © Monkey Business Images Ltd/Monkey Business/Getty Images.)

Every patient—or a legal representative for that patient, such as a parent or spouse—must give consent for surgery.

- Having a signed consent form on file protects not just the patient but also the surgeon and other staff, as well as the healthcare facility.
- There are different kinds of consent, depending on the treatment to be performed:
  - Consent for a medical or surgical treatment
  - Consent for the use of anesthesia

- Consent for the administration of blood products (members of some groups, notably the Jehovah's Witnesses religious sect, may refuse blood products)
- Consent to be sterilized
- Consent to undergo investigational methods
- Consent for disposal of any body parts or tissues that are removed
- Consent is obtained before any medications that might cloud the patient's judgment are administered.
- The surgeon obtains consent after carefully explaining, in language that the patient can understand, the procedure, its risks and likelihood of success, and any possible complications, as well as alternatives to the procedure. This allows the patient to give **informed consent**, making an educated decision to proceed.
- The patient must be a legal adult (age 18 years or older) to give consent, with some exceptions:
  - Children who have been granted legal responsibility for their own affairs (**emancipated minor**) may give consent.
  - A minor who has **given birth** may give consent.
- The consent form must be signed by the **patient, the surgeon, and a witness**, generally the patient's spouse or legal guardian (a parent or other person appointed by a court to manage the patient's affairs).
- Consent must be given willingly. Coercion or intimidation by the surgeon, by healthcare staff, or by the patient's family renders a patient's consent invalid.
- If a patient requires treatment but is not conscious, not mentally competent, or not of an age to legally grant consent and there is no way to reach a family member or guardian, the consent form is signed by **two consulting physicians** (not including the surgeon) **and the hospital administrator.**
- The time and date of the signatures must be recorded carefully to help cement the legality of the document.

Legal Proceedings

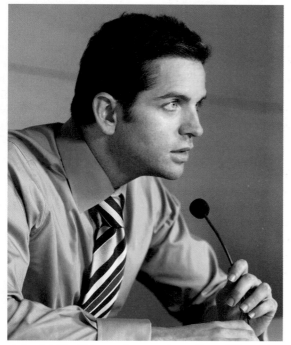

(Copyright © Mike Watson Images/moodboard/Getty Images.)

- Civil cases involve a **plaintiff** (the person or party that initiates a lawsuit to seek resolution) and a **defendant** (the person or party who is being sued.)
- Criminal cases involve the **state** (the local, state, or federal government), which pursues a case on behalf of its citizens; and a **defendant** (the person who has been charged with a crime).
- Occasionally you may be called upon, as a medical professional, to provide information, or **testify**, either during preparations for a legal case or when a case goes to court.
  - Testifying as part of the preparations for a trial is called giving a **deposition** or **being deposed.** A deposition may be requested by the plaintiff or state, by the defendant, or both. The information you provide may be recorded by a court reporter to construct a printed record, or you may be video- or audiotaped as you testify.
  - A judge may issue a **subpoena**, a ruling that compels a person to appear and testify at a trial. Subpoenas are also issued to force an institution or some other entity to provide requested documents.
  - You might also submit an **affidavit**, a sworn written statement that you provide voluntarily, to the court.
  - Whenever you are asked to testify, it is important to be as truthful as possible. Lying under oath, known as **perjury**, is considered a crime.
- In addition to lawsuits and criminal proceedings, the law allows people to specify how they want to be treated should they become incapable of making decisions about their health care. This is done through the use of legally binding documents called **advance directives.** There are several types:
  - A **living will** sets forth the treatments you do and do not want to have used to keep you alive—for instance, some people want to have cardiopulmonary resuscitation or mechanical ventilation performed, and others do not.
  - A **durable power of attorney for health care** specifies the person you want to make healthcare decisions on your behalf if you become unable to make them yourself.
- Some patients inform their medical providers that they want what is known as a do-not-resuscitate order, or **DNR.**
  - A DNR specifies that the patient wants the medical staff to **withhold** cardiopulmonary resuscitation (CPR) and/or mechanical ventilation in the event that he or she stops breathing or the heart ceases to beat.
  - A patient may request a DNR by asking medical staff to document his or her wishes **in the medical record** or by spelling it out **in an advance directive.**
  - However it is made, a DNR is a **legally binding** order.
  - A patient with a DNR on file may still undergo **medical treatment or surgery.**
  - A DNR may be revoked by the patient at any time.

ETHICS

Ethics is a topic that affects every human being on the planet but holds special significance for medical professionals. Broadly defined, ethics is the area of philosophy devoted to the study and classification of right and wrong.

For healthcare providers, ethics is a matter of always striving to do what is best for the patient. (Think back to the Latin phrases we discussed earlier in this chapter, specifically *aeger primo* ("The patient first") and *primum non nocere* ("Above all, do no harm").

Just about every healthcare discipline has a code of ethics or conduct that its members are expected to honor, and surgical technology is no exception (Box 6.2).

POLICIES AND PROCEDURES

All healthcare providers must follow local, state, and federal law, but they must also adhere to their healthcare institutions' **policies**. These rules and regulations, some of them based in law, are intended to keep patients and staff safe, streamline treatment, and help curb costs.

- Like other innovations in health care, modern safety mechanisms are a result of **evidence-based medicine**, in which data from scientific research, rather than anecdotal findings or tradition, are the basis for determining best practices.
- The Joint Commission (TJC) has issued a set of recommendations, called **Speak Up**, to help ensure that surgeries are conducted safely. Among these recommendations:
  - A **pre-procedure assessment** must be conducted to ensure that all supplies and equipment are available, that the appropriate procedure is being performed on the appropriate patient, and that all pertinent documents have been signed or are otherwise available.
  - The body part to undergo surgery must be **marked clearly** to prevent surgery on the wrong body part.
  - A **time-out**—a period during which all questions and concerns regarding a procedure are addressed (including a final verification that the right procedure is being performed on the right part of the right patient)—must be held by the surgical team (surgeon, nurse, surgical technologist, anesthesia provider, and any other staff) before any incision or other invasive procedure is begun. If more than one procedure is being performed, a time-out is held for each one.
- TJC also mandates that every **sentinel event**—any occurrence in a healthcare setting that is not related to a patient's illness but causes serious injury or the death of the patient—be reported to TJC and tracked in a database by the healthcare institution to make it easier to identify and address problems.
- The **Safe Medical Devices Act of 1990** is a federal law that requires facilities to report to the U.S. Department of Health and Human Services, the manufacturer, or both any case in which it is believed that a medical device has contributed to a patient's injury, illness, or death.
- As you've already seen in **Chapter 4: Aseptic Technique and Wound Management,** just about every hospital and surgical center has policies and procedures in place governing surgical counts.

CONCLUSION

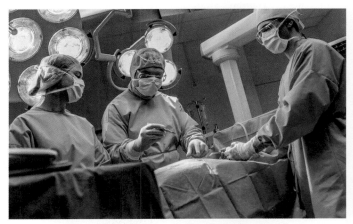

(Copyright © Simonkr/E+/Getty Images.)

Every member of the surgical team has a specific job, and as a surgical technologist, your job is much more than just passing instruments to the surgeon. You will be relied upon to bring your expertise in aseptic technique to the operating room and to serve, often, as a partner to the surgeon. Your reliability and professionalism will be crucial to the success of every procedure you attend.

Congratulations on completing this review of professionalism in surgical technology! If you feel ready, complete the chapter review questions and check your answers on the Evolve Resources site. If you think you might need a little more review, make your way back through the chapter, focusing on any weak areas.

REVIEW QUESTIONS

1. Surgical technologists are certified after successfully completing a surgical technology program accredited by the Commission on Accreditation of Allied Health Education Programs (CAAHEP) or the Accrediting Bureau of Health Education Schools (ABHES) and passing the national Certified Surgical Technologist (CST) examination administered by:
   a. LCCT
   b. NBSTSA
   c. ARC/STSA
   d. CAAHEP

2. This organization's primary purpose is ensuring that surgical technologists have the knowledge and skills to administer patient care of the highest quality. It is the principal provider, in conjunction with more than 40 state organizations, of continuing education for surgical technologists.
   a. AST
   b. ARC/STSA
   c. NBSTSA
   d. CAAHEP

3. Which of these statements is **not** true?
   a. Certification is not a permission to act but rather a statement of completion or qualification.
   b. Certification is a permission to do something that is otherwise forbidden.
   c. Certification is a statement or declaration that one has completed a course of study, passed an examination, or otherwise met specified criteria for certification.
   d. Certification is based on the premise that there is a right to work.

4. The willingness to be held liable for one's own actions in providing health care to the patient and not hesitating to admit a break in aseptic technique is:
   a. Surgical procedure
   b. Surgical intervention
   c. Surgical plan
   d. Surgical conscience

5. Which of these statements regarding the Association of Surgical Technologists' Professional Code of Conduct is true?
   a. Provide need to know basis treatment to all members and staff of the association in terms of professional rights and responsibilities
   b. Adhere to the bylaws and policies and procedures of the association at all times when not conducting business in any capacity
   c. To use coercive means or promise special treatment in order to influence professional decisions of fellow members
   d. Honestly represent the association or the constituent division with which that person is affiliated and shall refrain from expressing personal opinions that are contradictory to the association's positions.

6. Maslow's Hierarchy of Needs is divided into main types of needs:
   a. Basic and growth
   b. Physiological and self-actualization
   c. Growth and love
   d. Self-esteem and safety

7. Good group dynamics play a significant role in education and group learning by:
   a. Enhancing interpersonal relations and communication skills
   b. Fostering critical thinking
   c. Improving social interaction
   d. Clarifying doubts

8. What is the term for the messages we send to express ideas and opinions through the use of body language, facial expressions, gestures, touch or contact, signs, symbols, pictures, objects, and other visual aids?
   a. Eye contact communication
   b. General communication
   c. Verbal communication
   d. Nonverbal communication

9. The ability to explain your ideas clearly through use of the spoken word and to listen carefully to other people represents good:
   a. Nonverbal communication
   b. Verbal communication
   c. General communication
   d. Sign language communication

10. This theory of development holds that achieving a balance between autonomy and shame and doubt leads to the development of will, the ability to act with intention, within reason and limits.
    a. Erikson's
    b. Sigmund's
    c. Einstein's
    d. Newton's

7

Perioperative Case Management

OUTLINE

In this chapter, we'll review various surgeries with which you need to be familiar for your certification exam.

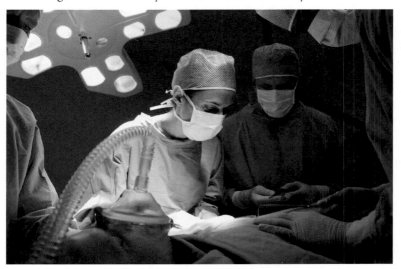

(Copyright © Monkey Business Images/Monkey Business/Getty Images.)

GENERAL SURGERY

This section is divided into three parts:
- Abdominal wall procedures
- Abdominal contents procedures
- Breast procedures

Abdominal Wall Surgeries

Surgeries of the abdominal wall are all types of *herniorrhaphy*. As you have probably deduced from your past studies and your reading of **Chapter 1: Medical Terminology**, this term means "suturing of a hernia"—hernia repair. A hernia is a protrusion of an organ through a weakened spot in the abdominal wall nearby; the defect may be congenital or acquired (usually as a result of blunt trauma) (Fig. 7.1). There are several kinds of herniorrhaphy procedures; they may be performed laparoscopically or as open surgeries.

Procedures
- Direct inguinal hernia repair
- Indirect inguinal hernia repair
- Pantaloon hernia repair (repair of direct and indirect hernias at the same site in the same surgery)
- Hiatal hernia repair
- Incisional hernia repair (a.k.a. ventral hernia repair)
- Incarcerated (a.k.a irreducible) hernia repair
- Strangulated hernia repair

Basic Laparoscopic Equipment Required
- Light cord
- Camera
- Insufflation tubing (for introduction of CO_2 gas to induce pneumoperitoneum)
- Trocars (surgeon's preference as to type)
- Laparoscopy instruments
- General surgery major soft instruments

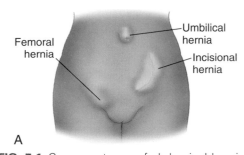

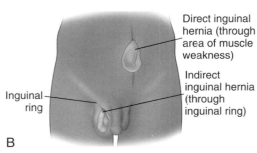

FIG. 7.1 Common types of abdominal hernias. **A,** *Umbilical* hernias result from a weakness in the abdominal wall around the umbilicus. An *incisional* hernia is herniation through inadequately healed surgery. In a *femoral* hernia, a loop of intestine descends through the femoral canal into the groin (femoral means "pertaining to the thigh"). **B,** *Inguinal* hernias are of two types. A *direct* hernia occurs through an area of weakness in the abdominal wall. In an *indirect* hernia, a loop of intestine descends through the inguinal canal, an opening in the abdominal wall for passage of the spermatic cord in males, and a ligament of the uterus in females. (From Leonard PC: Quick & easy medical terminology, ed 8, St Louis, 2017, Elsevier.)

Other Instrument/Equipment Required

- General surgery major soft tissue instrumentation (if incision is extended or any bowel is involved)
- Synthetic mesh (placed, in most procedures, over the defect; may or may not be sutured or stapled into place)
- Electrosurgical unit
- Harmonic scalpel (may be needed)

Basic Anatomy Involved

The surgeon must make his or her way through quite a few layers of abdominal wall (Fig. 7.2).

- Skin
- Fascia of Camper (superficial fatty layer of the subcutaneous tissue)
- Fascia of Scarpa (deep membranous layer of the subcutaneous tissue)

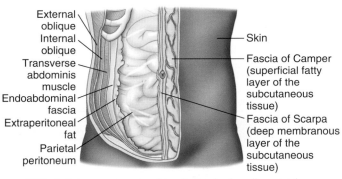

FIG. 7.2 Layers involved in abdominal wall surgeries.

- External oblique
- Internal oblique
- Transverse abdominis muscle
- Endoabdominal fascia
- Extraperitoneal fat
- Parietal peritoneum

Additional Facts to Remember

- A **Penrose drain** is used to retract the spermatic cord in male patients.
- Direct and indirect inguinal hernia repairs both involve **mesh repair with sutures or staples**, as does incisional/ventral hernia repair.
- Hiatal hernia repair (laparoscopic Nissen fundoplication) may be converted to **laparotomy** if:
  - The patient is obese
  - The patient has a short esophagus
  - The patient has a history of surgery in the upper abdominal area
- Two different laparoscopic approaches are used to correct direct inguinal hernia:
  - TAPP (transabdominal preperitoneal procedure), in which pneumoperitoneum is established
  - TEP (total extraperitoneal procedure), in which a balloon expander is inserted into the incision and used to instill air or normal saline solution (no pneumoperitoneum)

Mapping

Here's how hernia procedures look once they've been mapped:

SURGICAL MAPPING

Direct inguinal hernia (acquired)

Instruments	Important Anatomy Involved	Pathophysiology
General surgery minor; instruments Soft tissue/laparoscopic instruments	Hesselbach triangle (between rectus abdominis muscle, inguinal ligament, and inferior epigastric artery)	Heavy lifting Chronic cough Constipation
Microbiology/Wound Classification	**Skin Prep/Incision/Patient position**	**Pharmacology**
Class I (clean)	*Prep:* Midchest to pubis symphysis (may be extended to midthigh) *Incision:* oblique *Position:* supine	Antibiotic irrigation Lidocaine (before incision) or marcaine (post-op) or 50/50 combo

SURGICAL MAPPING

Indirect inguinal hernia (congenital)

Instruments	Important Anatomy Involved	Pathophysiology
General surgery minor instruments Soft tissue/laparoscopic instruments	Peritoneal sac protrudes through internal inguinal ring and passes through inguinal canal; scrotum may be involved	Congenital defect in fascial floor of inguinal canal
Microbiology/Wound Classification	**Skin Prep/Incision/Patient position**	**Pharmacology**
Class I (clean)	*Prep:* midchest to pubis symphysis (may be extended to midthigh) *Incision:* oblique *Position:* supine	Antibiotic irrigation Lidocaine (before incision) or marcaine (post-op)

SURGICAL MAPPING

Incisional/ventral hernia repair (traumatic)

Instruments	Important Anatomy Involved	Pathophysiology
General surgery major; soft tissue instruments (if incision is extended or any bowel is involved)	Abdominal contents protrude through peritoneal fascia	Previous surgical incision
Microbiology/Wound Classification	**Skin Prep/Incision/Patient position**	**Pharmacology**
C ass II (clean contaminated); bowel may be strangulated, requiring extension of procedure to bowel resection	*Prep:* midchest to pubis symphysis (may be extended to midthigh) *Incision:* based on previous surgical incision *Position:* supine	Antibiotic irrigation Lidocaine (before incision) or marcaine (post-op)

SURGICAL MAPPING

Hiatal hernia

Instruments	Important Anatomy Involved	Pathophysiology
Laparoscopic instrumentation; Maloney dilator (inserted by anesthesiologist)	Portion of stomach protrudes through hiatus of diaphragm. On dissection of left pillar of crus, vagus nerve is identified	Weakening of hiatal opening
Microbiology/Wound Classification	**Skin Prep/Incision/Patient position**	**Pharmacology**
Class I (clean)	*Prep:* midchest to pubis symphysis (may be extended to midthigh) *Incision:* midline *Position:* supine	Lidocaine or marcaine

SURGICAL MAPPING

TAPP (transabdominal preperitoneal procedure; pneumoperitoneum)

Instruments	Important Anatomy Involved	Pathophysiology
Laparoscopic instrumentation	Hesselbach triangle (between rectus abdominis muscle, inguinal ligament, and inferior epigastric artery)	Heavy lifting Chronic cough Constipation
Microbiology/Wound Classification	**Skin Prep/Incision/Patient position**	**Pharmacology**
>Class I (clean)	*Prep:* midchest to pubis symphysis (may be extended to midthigh) *Incision:* transverse, directly above hernia space *Position:* supine	Lidocaine, marcaine , or 50/50 combo

SURGICAL MAPPING

TEP (total extraperitoneal procedure; balloon expander with air or saline)

Instruments	Important Anatomy Involved	Pathophysiology
Laparoscopic instrumentation	Hesselbach triangle	Heavy lifting Chronic cough Constipation
Microbiology/Wound Classification	**Skin Prep/Incision/Patient position**	**Pharmacology**
Class I (clean)	*Prep:* midchest to pubis symphysis (may be extended to midthigh) *Incision:* periumbilical, through rectus sheath *Position:* supine	Lidocaine, marcaine, or 50/50 combo

Now, you try mapping the remaining procedures, using the template available on the Evolve Resources site.
- Pantaloon hernia repair
- Incarcerated hernia repair
- Strangulated hernia repair

Abdominal Contents Surgeries
Procedures
- Gastrectomy
- Roux-en-Y
- Billroth I (gastroduodenal anastomosis)

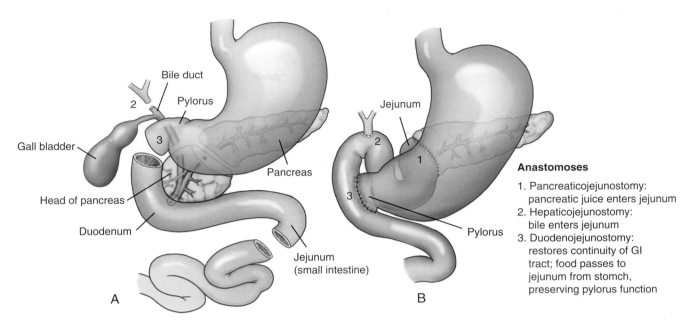

Anastomoses

1. Pancreaticojejunostomy: pancreatic juice enters jejunum
2. Hepaticojejunostomy: bile enters jejunum
3. Duodenojejunostomy: restores continuity of GI tract; food passes to jejunum from stomch, preserving pylorus function

FIG. 7.3 Whipple procedure (a.k.a. radical pancreaticoduodenectomy).

- Billroth II (gastrojejunal anastomosis)
- Colon resection
- Sigmoidectomy
- Liver resection
- Splenectomy
- Whipple procedure (pancreaticoduodenectomy; Fig. 7.3)
- Cholecystectomy

Additional Facts to Remember
- The steps in the Whipple procedure are:
  - Anastomosis of the proximal end of the jejunum to the pancreatic body

- Anastomosis of common bile duct (CBD) to jejunum in an end-to-end technique
- Anastomosis of distal stomach to the jejunum in an end-to-end technique
- Preoperative site selection for stoma creation is not possible; a site is selected intraoperatively at a point below the costal margin, above the belt line and appropriate lateral edge of the rectus abdominis muscle.

Mapping
Here you can see how two of these procedures map:

SURGICAL MAPPING

Whipple procedure (pancreaticoduodenum)

Instruments	Important Anatomy Involved	Pathophysiology
General surgery major instrumentation	Distal stomach	Cancer of head of pancreas
Book Walter retractor	Duodenum	Incision
Vascular instrumentation	Jejunum	
	Common bile duct	
	Head of pancreas	

Microbiology/Wound Classification	Skin Prep/Incision/Patient position	Pharmacology
If there no bowel or biliary tract spillage, class II (clean contaminated)	*Prep:* midchest to pubis symphysis (extended to midthigh)	General anesthesia
If bowel or biliary tract spillage, class III (contaminated)	*Incision:* upper transverse, paramedian or bilateral subcostal	
	Position: supine	

NORMAL ANATOMY

In a **modified radical mastectomy**, breast tissue, nipple, and lymph nodes are removed, but muscles are left intact.

To drainage device

Axillary dissection

In a **simple mastectomy**, breast tissue and (usually) nipple are removed, but lymph nodes are left intact.

In a **lumpectomy with lymph node dissection**, only the tumor and lymph nodes are removed. Other tissue is left intact.

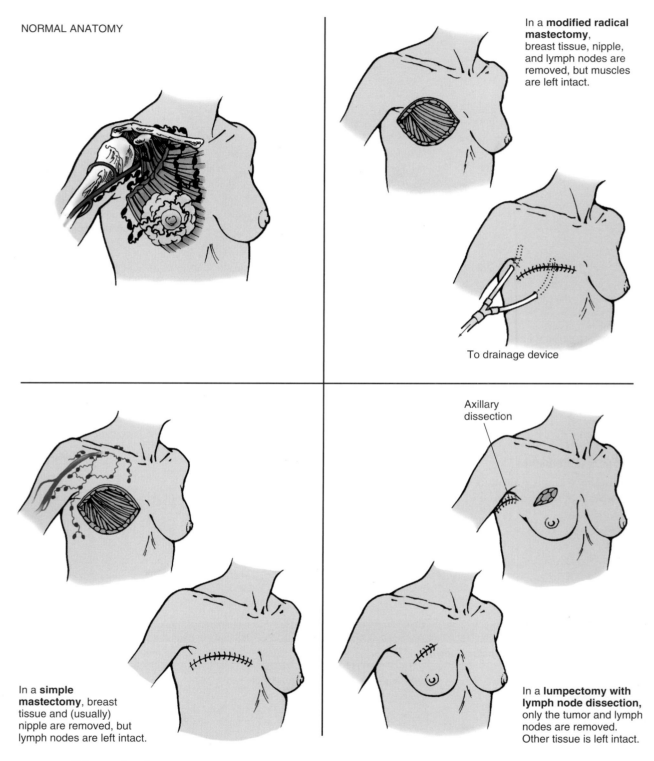

FIG. 7.4 Surgical management of breast cancer. (From Ignatavicius DD, Workman ML: *Medical-surgical nursing: patient-centered collaborative care*, ed 7, St Louis, 2013, Saunders.)

SURGICAL MAPPING

Cholecystectomy (open or laparoscopic)

Instruments	Important Anatomy Involved	Pathophysiology
Open: General surgery major instrumentation Book Walter retractor *Laparoscopic:* Laparoscopic instrumentation Clip appliers	Gallbladder Cystic duct Cystic artery Liver	Cholelithiasis

Microbiology/Wound Classification	Skin Prep/Incision/Patient position	Pharmacology
Salmonella typhi *Laparoscopic:* class I (clean) *With cholangiogram:* class II (clean contaminated) *If spillage from duct:* class III (contaminated)	*Prep:* midchest to pubis symphysis; extended to midthigh *Open incision:* right subcostal (Kocher) *Laparoscopic incision:* umbilical *Position:* supine	General anesthesia *With cholangiogram:* contrast medium (Hypaque)

Mapping

Use the template available on the Evolve Resources site to try your hand at mapping the remaining procedures in this category:

- Gastrectomy
- Roux-en-Y
- Billroth I (gastroduodenal anastomosis)
- Billroth II (gastrojejunal anastomosis)
- Colon resection
- Sigmoidectomy
- Liver resection
- Splenectomy

Breast Surgeries

See Fig. 7.4.

Procedures

- Needle localization
- Breast biopsy
- Sentinel node biopsy
- Mastectomy
  - Total or simple
    - The entire breast is removed.
    - The axillary lymph nodes are left intact.
    - The muscle of the chest wall is preserved.
  - Modified
    - The entire breast is removed.
    - The axillary lymph nodes are removed.
    - The muscle of the chest wall is preserved.
  - Radical
    - The entire breast is removed.
    - The axillary lymph nodes are removed.
    - The muscle of the chest wall is removed as well.

Additional Facts to Remember

- Whenever mastectomy will be followed by reconstruction, the surgical technologist in the scrub role (STSR) should have **two setups** ready. This helps prevent inadvertent **seeding** (spread of cancer cells on contaminated instruments).

- For sentinel node biopsy, the surgeon uses **isosulfan blue dye** (Lymphazurin) with a radioactive colloid and a gamma probe to identify the lymphatic drainage of a tumor.
  - Remember the **rule of fives**:
    - **Five milliliters** of dye is injected.
    - Dye is injected into **five** sites.
    - The injection sites span a **5-cm** diameter.
    - The site is massaged for **5 minutes**.
- The wound is irrigated with **warm sterile water.** Why? The warm water is absorbed by cells, including cancerous ones that may be present. As a result of osmosis, the cells burst (hypotonic solution).
- Most tissue specimens taken for breast biopsy or mastectomy are removed **en bloc** (in one piece).

Mapping

Let's map a mastectomy procedure:

SURGICAL MAPPING

Modified mastectomy

Instruments	Important Anatomy Involved	Pathophysiology
General surgery Major soft instrumentation with additional Allis and Adair clamps and various sizes of rakes	Breast tissue Axillary lymph nodes Chest wall muscle	Cancer

Microbiology/Wound Classification	Skin Prep/Incision/ Patient position	Pharmacology
No indigenous microorganisms in breast other than cancer cells Class I (clean)	*Prep:* from site of incision to neck, medial to sternum toward mid-abdomen, laterally to axilla and arm to elbow *Incision:* elliptical transverse *Position:* supine	General anesthesia

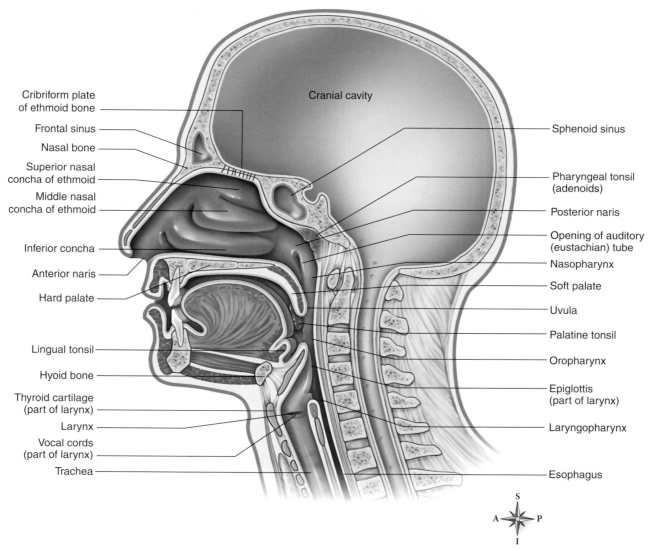

FIG. 7.5 Sagittal section of the head and neck. The nasal septum has been removed, exposing the right lateral wall of the nasal cavity so that the nasal conchae can be seen. Note also the divisions of the pharynx and the position of the tonsils. (From Patton KT, Thibodeau GA: The human body in health & disease, ed 6, St Louis, 2014, Mosby.)

OK, now it's your turn! Go ahead and map the remaining procedures, using the template available on the Evolve Resources site:
- Breast biopsy
- Sentinel node biopsy
- Total (simple) mastectomy
- Radical mastectomy

ENT (OTORHINOLARYNGOLOGIC) SURGERIES

ENT surgeries involve structures of the ears, nose, throat, head, and neck (Fig. 7.5). This section is divided into three parts:
- Ear procedures
- Nasal procedures
- Throat procedures

Ear Procedures
Procedures
- Myringotomy

- Tympanoplasty
- Mastoidectomy
- Stapedectomy
- Cochlear implant

Additional Facts to Remember
- A **microscope** is used for all ear cases.
- The middle and inner ear are **sterile** (indigenous microorganisms present), so all such cases are categorized as **class I (clean).**
- In ENT surgery, **epinephrine** is used in conjunction with any local anesthesia because it prolongs the action of the anesthetic agent and because, as a vasoconstrictor, it minimizes bleeding.

Mapping
Here's how one ear procedure maps:

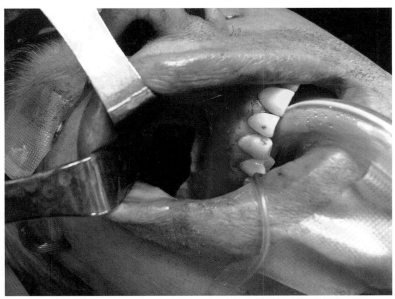

FIG. 7.6 Caldwell-Luc operation. (From Ignatavicius DD, Workman ML: *Medical surgical nursing: critical thinking for collaborative care*, ed 5, St Louis, 2006, Mosby.)

SURGICAL MAPPING

Myringotomy

Instruments	Important Anatomy Involved	Pathophysiology
ENT tray: Farrior speculum Frazier suction Myringotomy knife Alligator forceps	Tympanic membrane	Effusion in middle ear, caused by inflammation of mucosa

Microbiology/Wound Classification	Skin Prep/Incision/Patient position	Pharmacology
Indigenous flora present in external ear *Pseudomonas aeruginosa* and *Staphylococcus aureus* Class III (dirty)	*Prep:* none *Incision:* vertical, into tympanic membrane *Position:* supine head supported on doughnut headrest	General anesthesia given by mask (short procedure) Hydrogen peroxide to loosen any hard wax (cerumen) before incision

Go ahead and use the template available on the Evolve Resources site to map the remaining procedures:

- Tympanoplasty
- Mastoidectomy
- Stapedectomy
- Cochlear implant

Nasal Procedures

Procedures

- Septoplasty
- Turbinectomy
- Nasal polypectomy
- Choanal atresia repair
- FESS (functional endoscopic sinus surgery)
- Caldwell-Luc antrostomy (a.k.a. nasal antrostomy; Fig. 7.6)
- Rhinoplasty

Additional Facts to Remember

- **Cocaine 4%** is used as a topical anesthetic; it also acts as a vasoconstrictor.
- Any surgery performed through the nose is considered **nonsterile**, with a wound classification of class III (contaminated).
- **Repair of choanal atresia** (congenital absence of an opening into the nasopharynx) is performed in pediatric patients. The condition is usually suspected if an **8F catheter** cannot be inserted where the opening should be. A powered burr or microdebrider is used to make the repair.
- In **Caldwell-Luc antrostomy**, the incision is made above the canine and second molar.
- It is important to identify and avoid damaging the **infraorbital nerve**, which could result in blindness or infraorbital neuralgia, a painful disorder that may be misdiagnosed as migraine.
- **Absorbable sutures** are used in these procedures.

Mapping

Here's the mapping on a couple of nasal surgeries.

SURGICAL MAPPING

Rhinoplasty

Instruments	Important Anatomy Involved	Pathophysiology
Basic nasal instrumentation	Nasal septum Ethmoid and vomer bones	Deformity of external nose (traumatic, congenital, or disease-related)

Microbiology/ Wound Classification	Skin Prep/Incision/ Patient position	Pharmacology
Class III (dirty)	*Prep:* none *Incision:* at nasal skin *Position:* usually supine with neck hyperextended (tilted with shoulder roll)	Lidocaine with epinephrine, oxymetazoline (Afrin), or cocaine

SURGICAL MAPPING

FESS (functional endoscopic sinus surgery)

Instruments	Important Anatomy Involved	Pathophysiology
Basic nasal instrumentation Endoscopic instruments Sinus scope (4- or 5-mm with 0, 30, 70, and 120-degree lenses) Suction irrigation Antifog for lenses Navigational system that uses CT images	Paranasal sinuses (frontal, ethmoid, sphenoid, maxillary)	Congenital defect, chronic sinusitis, other sinus disorders

Microbiology/ Wound Classification	Skin Prep/Incision/ Patient position	Pharmacology
Class III (dirty)	*Prep:* none *Position:* usually supine with neck hyperextended (tilted with shoulder roll)	Lidocaine with epinephrine, or oxymetazoline (Afrin), or cocaine

Ready to map the remaining procedures? They are:

- Septoplasty
- Turbinectomy
- Polypectomy
- Choanal atresia repair
- Caldwell-Luc antrostomy (a.k.a. nasal antrostomy)
  Use the template available on the Evolve Resources site.

Throat Surgeries
Procedures

- Tonsillectomy
- Laryngectomy
- Adenoidectomy
- UPPP (uvulopalatopharyngoplasty)
- Radical neck dissection with mandibulectomy (removal of mandible) or glossectomy (removal of tongue)
- Tracheostomy/tracheotomy
- TMJ (temporomandibular joint) arthroscopy
- Parotidectomy (Fig. 7.7)
- Thyroidectomy

Additional ENT Facts to Remember

- **Tonsillectomy/adenoidectomy** is performed in conjunction with UPPP if the tonsils or adenoids are hypertrophied.
- UPPP is performed to treat **obstructive sleep apnea**; it is reasoned that removal of this tissue will widen the patient's airway, making breathing easier.
- Radical neck dissection is mainly performed to treat **metastatic squamous cell carcinoma. Mandibulectomy and tracheostomy** are performed in conjunction with this procedure. **Two setups and two teams** are required: one for radical neck dissection (sterile part, class I [clean]) and the other for oromaxillofacial surgery (nonsterile part, class III [dirty]). Most cases of radical neck dissection involve a combination of glossectomy and mandibulectomy.
- **TMJ arthroscopy** is similar in concept to any other arthroscopic procedure (discussed later in chapter). **Lactated Ringer solution** is used for irrigation. Wound classification is **class I (clean).**
- During parotidectomy, it is important to identify and avoid injuring the **facial nerve** (cranial nerve VII). This nerve controls facial expression; injury results in facial nerve palsy.
- Use of a **harmonic scalpel** is preferred for removal of a diseased thyroid gland because it is as safe as conventional methods of hemostasis and quicker because the need for repetitive "clip, cut, tie" routines is eliminated.
- A handheld **Green loop retractor and Weitlaner clamp** are part of the normal instrument tray for this procedure.
- A transverse incision **following the Langer line** is performed in radical neck dissection.
- The **superior and recurrent laryngeal nerves** are important surgical landmarks to be preserved during throat surgeries. They innervate the vocal cord.
- For blunt dissection in throat surgery, **cotton peanuts** (Kitners) are used.
- The superior thyroid artery is **double-clamped, divided, and ligated.**

Mapping

Now we'll map one of the most commonly performed throat surgeries.

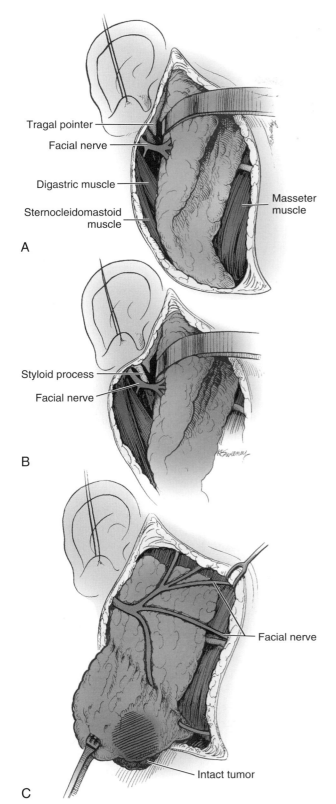

FIG. 7.7 Parotidectomy. Operative technique for parotidectomy. **A,** Blunt dissection of parotid gland from external auditory canal cartilage exposes tragal pointer. Facial nerve lies approximately 1 cm deep and slightly anteroinferior to pointer and 6 to 8 mm deep to tympanomastoid suture line. **B,** Facial nerve exits stylomastoid foramen to run anteriorly between styloid process and attachment of digastric muscle to digastric ridge. **C,** Nearly completed process with tumor within intact superficial parotidectomy specimen. (From Cummings CW et al: *Otolaryngology: head and neck surgery,* ed 3, St Louis, 1993, Mosby.)

SURGICAL MAPPING

Tonsillectomy/ adenoidectomy

Instruments	Important Anatomy Involved	Pathophysiology
Tonsillectomy/adenoidectomy instrument tray	Palatine and pharyngeal tonsils	Chronic tonsillitis Peritonsillar abscess due to failed antibiotic therapy

Microbiology/Wound Classification	Skin Prep/Incision/ Patient position	Pharmacology
Streptococcus pneumoniae *Haemophilus influenzae* *Neisseria* species Aerobic streptococci Class III (dirty)	*Prep:* none *Incision:* into palatine/ pharyngeal tonsils *Position:* supine with neck hyperextended	General anesthesia

SURGICAL MAPPING

Thyroidectomy

Instruments	Important Anatomy Involved	Pathophysiology
Thyroidectomy instrument set Lahey thyroid clamp Green loop retractor Weitlaner clamp	Thyroid gland Parathyroid gland Recurrent laryngeal nerve	Hyperthyroidism Thyrotoxicosis thyroid Carcinoma

Microbiology/ Wound Classification	Skin Prep/Incision/ Patient position	Pharmacology
No indigenous microorganisms in thyroid Class I (clean)	*Prep:* point of chin to midchest *Incision:* transverse along Langer lines *Position:* supine with neck hyperextended	General anesthesia

OK, it's your turn! Use the template available on the Evolve Resources site to map the remaining procedures:

- UPPP (uvulopalatopharyngoplasty)
- Radical neck dissection with mandibulectomy or glossectomy
- Tracheostomy/tracheotomy
- TMJ (temporomandibular joint) arthroscopy
- Parotidectomy

OB/GYN SURGERY

OB/GYN surgery consists of procedures involving the female reproductive organs (Fig. 7.8), both in pregnancy (obstetric, OB) and situations of general gynecology (GYN).

- Obstetric procedures
- Gynecologic abdominal contents procedures
- Vaginal procedures

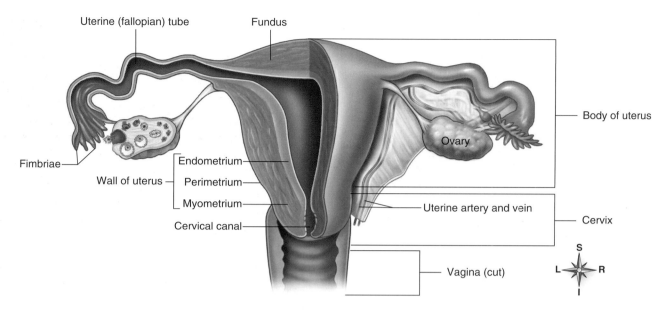

Uterine (fallopian) tube

Fundus

Body of uterus

Ovary

Fimbriae

Endometrium

Wall of uterus

Perimetrium

Myometrium

Uterine artery and vein

Cervix

Cervical canal

Vagina (cut)

FIG. 7.8 Internal female reproductive organs. Posterior view. Diagram shows left side of uterus and upper portion of the vagina and the left uterine tube and ovary in a frontal section. The broad ligament has been removed from the posterior surface of the uterus and adjacent structures. (From Patton KT, Thibodeau GA: The human body in health & disease, ed 6, St Louis, 2014, Mosby.)

Obstetric Surgeries

Procedures

- Cesarean section
- Cervical cerclage
- Vaginal delivery

Basic Anatomy Involved

- Uterus
- Bladder
- Round ligament
- Broad ligament
- Cardinal ligament
- Uterosacral ligament

Additional Facts to Remember

- In most OB/GYN procedures, a **Foley or straight catheter** will be inserted beforehand to decompress the bladder and help prevent injury.

  #### C-section or Vaginal Delivery
- Remember that **failure to progress** is the primary indicator for C-section.
- In a C-section, **four surgical counts** are taken:
  - Before skin incision
  - Before closure of the uterus
  - Before closure of the peritoneum (abdominal cavity)
  - Before closure of the skin
- The **bladder** is freed from the uterus before an incision is made into the uterus.
- The umbilical cord is cut either with **Lister bandage scissors** or **curved Mayo scissors.**
- Umbilical cord blood may be collected for **cord blood gas determination.** Why? Umbilical cord pH and blood gas values provide valuable information regarding an infant's metabolic condition at birth; base excess determination quantifies

the magnitude of perinatal hypoxia/asphyxia and metabolic acidosis, the putative risk factor for central neurological injury

- A **De Lee suction catheter** is used to suction meconium-stained amniotic fluid. Before or during labor, the fetus sometimes passes meconium (fetal stool) into the amniotic sac. The reason is not clearly understood, but this phenomenon is thought to be related to fetal distress in some babies. The thick meconium mixes with the amniotic fluid and then swallowed and breathed into the airway by the fetus. As the neonate takes the first breaths after delivery, meconium particles may enter the airway and be aspirated deep into the lungs.
- The **placenta** is placed in a large basin and passed off to the circulating nurse, who will check for evidence of abnormality, such as infection or chronic blood deprivation, and determine whether the placenta is whole or shows any meconium discoloration.

Cervical Cerclage (Shirodkar and McDonald Procedures)

- Shirodkar: In this procedure, a suture is used to close the internal os in a pregnant woman whose cervix has failed to retain previous pregnancies. The sutures are passed through the walls of the cervix so they're not exposed. In most cases, a cesarean section will eventually be performed.
- McDonald: The internal os is sutured after the lower part has already started to efface (Fig. 7.9). Sutures are usually placed between 16 and 18 weeks of pregnancy and removed around the 37th week.
- These procedures are performed during the **second or third trimester** because the cervix tends to dilate spontaneously at this time, possibly resulting in spontaneous abortion.
- The procedure may be performed one of two ways:
  - In **transvaginal cerclage** (TVC), a band of synthetic Mersilene tape is placed around the proximal cervix through the vagina, and paracervical tissue is sutured with 2-0 or 3-0 synthetic absorbable sutures.

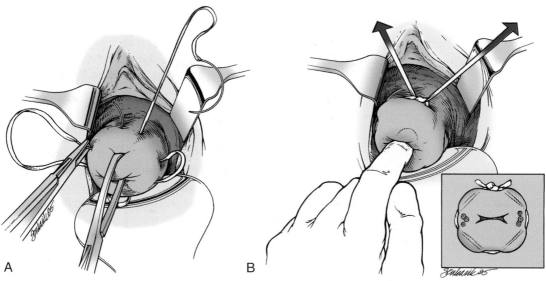

FIG. 7.9 Placement of sutures for McDonald cerclage. **A,** Double-headed Mersilene band with four bites in the cervix, avoiding the vessels. **B,** The suture is placed high up in the cervix, close to the cervicovaginal junction, approximately at the level of the internal os. (From Gabbe SG, et al: Obstetrics: normal and problem pregnancies, ed 7, Philadelphia, 2017, Elsevier.)

- In **transabdominal cerclage** (TAC), Mersilene tape (suture) is placed at the internal os after a short suprapubic incision is made. C-section is required for delivery.

Mapping

Here you can see how two commonly performed procedures, the cesarean section and cervical cerclage, look when they're mapped:

SURGICAL MAPPING

Cesarean section

Instruments	Important Anatomy Involved	Pathophysiology
C-section tray	Uterus	Failure to progress
Fetal monitor	Bladder	STD
Bulb syringe (for infant's airway)		Prior surgery
Cord blood container		Obstruction of birth canal
Radiant heater for infant warming bed		Placenta previa and abruption
Foley catheter (inserted if not already in place)		Presence of TAC band to prevent spontaneous abortion (cerclage)

Microbiology/ Wound Classification	Skin Prep/Incision/ Patient position	Pharmacology
Class I (clean)	*Prep:* abdominal prep plus vagina/inner thighs *Incision:* Pfannenstiel (low transverse) *Position:* supine position with roll under right hip to prevent uterine pressure on vena cava	Oxytocin (given by anesthesiologist to stimulate uterine contractions)

SURGICAL MAPPING

Cervical cerclage

Instruments	Important Anatomy Involved	Pathophysiology
D&C tray	Uterus	Incompetent cervix
Mersilene tape	Cervix	
	External cervical os	
	Internal cervical os	

Microbiology/ Wound Classification	Skin Prep/Incision/ Patient position	Pharmacology
Indigenous microorganisms of vagina (*Lactobacillus*) Class II (clean contaminated)	*Prep:* gentle vaginal prep, including inner thighs *Position:* lithotomy	Spinal, general or epidural anesthesia

Ready to map the remaining OB/GYN procedure? Use the template available on the Evolve Resources site.
- Vaginal delivery

Gynecologic Abdominal Contents Procedures

These procedures involve the uterus, fallopian tube, ovary, or some combination thereof. They may be performed as open surgeries or laparoscopically, depending on the procedure.

Laparoscopic Surgeries

Procedures
- Gynecologic laparoscopy
  - Tubal sterilization
  - Resection of ectopic pregnancy
  - Salpingectomy
  - Oophorectomy

- Myomectomy
- Tuboplasty
- LAVH (laparoscopically assisted vaginal hysterectomy)
- Bilateral salpingoophorectomy

Equipment

- Light cord
- Camera
- Insufflation tubing
- Trocars
- Laparoscopic instruments
- Minor soft instruments

Additional Facts to Remember

- In all GYN laparoscopic procedures, it is important to have a GYN major tray available along with other accessory supplies in case the surgeon decides to perform an open surgery.

Open Surgeries

Procedures

- TAH (total abdominal hysterectomy)

Radical hysterectomy (Fig. 7.10) is the removal of the ovaries, fallopian tubes, uterus, upper third of the vagina, and associated lymph nodes.

- Vaginal hysterectomy is removal of the uterus by way of a vaginal approach. It's ideal for the patient with a prolapsed uterus.
- Pelvic exenteration

Equipment

- GYN major instruments
- Retractors (see Chapter 3, Table 3-1)

Additional Facts to Remember

- In TAH and LAVH, a Foley or straight catheter will be inserted before the procedure to decompress the bladder and help prevent injury.
- When the final dissection is being made along the vaginal cuff to free the uterus in TAH, instruments that project into the vagina (e.g., Allis clamps) are considered contaminated and must be isolated.

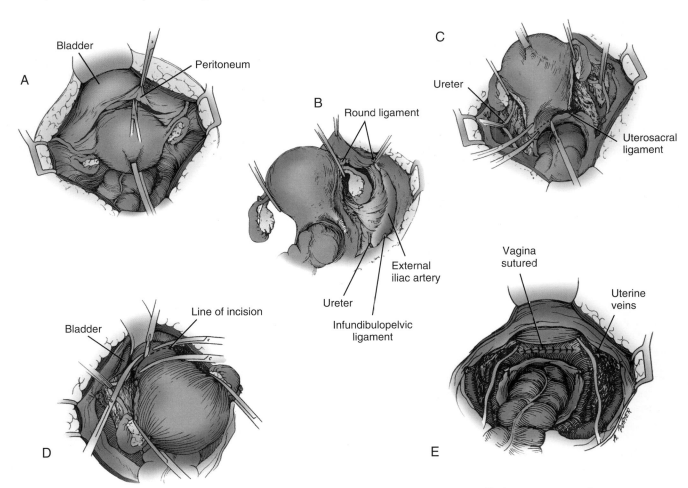

FIG. 7.10 Wertheim radical hysterectomy. **A,** With upward traction applied on uterus, peritoneum is incised from round ligament to round ligament. **B,** Right round and infundibulopelvic ligaments are ligated and cut, thus exposing right external iliac artery. **C,** Uterus is held upward and forward, exposing cul-de-sac, which is incised as shown by dotted line. **D,** After dissection is completed, vagina is doubly clamped preparatory to transection, after which entire specimen is lifted out en bloc. **E,** Vagina is closed. Peritoneum remains to be reperitonealized. (From Rothrock JC, Alexander SM: Alexander's surgical procedures, ed 1, St. Louis, 2012, Mosby.)

Mapping

Here's how total abdominal hysterectomy looks when mapped:

SURGICAL MAPPING

TAH (total abdominal hysterectomy), open or laparoscopic

Instruments	Important Anatomy Involved	Pathophysiology
GYN major instrumentation: O'Sullivan- O'Connor retractor Heaney clamps Jorgenson scissors *If laparoscopic:* Laparoscopic instrumentation Endoscopic stapler	Uterus Bladder Ureters Uterine ligaments	Uterine fibroids Cancer Endometriosis Abnormal uterine bleeding

Microbiology/ Wound Classification	Skin Prep/Incision/ Patient position	Pharmacology
No indigenous microorganisms in the uterus Class I (clean)	*Prep:* Midchest to pubis symphysis, extended to midthigh *Incision:* Pfannenstiel *Position:* supine **If laparoscopic:** *Incision:* umbilical *Position:* lithotomy	Warm normal saline General anesthesia

Go ahead and try to map the remaining procedures, using the template on the Evolve Resources site:

- Tuboplasty
- Tubal sterilization
- GYN laparoscopy
- Resection of ectopic pregnancy
- Myomectomy
- Pelvic exenteration
- Salpingectomy
- Oophorectomy

Vaginal Procedures
Procedures

- Marsupialization of abscessed Bartholin gland (Fig. 7.11)
- Hysteroscopy
- Anterior (cystocele) and posterior (rectocele) colporrhaphy
- Dilation & curettage (D&C)
- Suction D&C
- Labiaplasty
- Vulvectomy

Basic Hysteroscopy Equipment Required

- Light cord
- Camera
- Irrigation tubing
- Trocars
- Hysteroscopic instruments
- D&C instruments
- Fluid (medium for distention)
- Allen or candy cane stirrups for lithotomy position

Additional Facts to Remember

- Marsupialization of a Bartholin gland consists of incison, opening (like a kangaroo's pouch), and drainage of the gland, followed by suturing to keep the incision open and permit healing by granulation from the base of the pouch.
- Two types of specimens may be obtained during D&C: endometrial and endocervical.
- A **red rubber Robinson straight catheter** is used to decompress the bladder and help prevent injury.
- A **pudendal block**—injection of anesthetic into the pudendal canal, where the pudendal nerve is located—provides quick pain relief and blockage of sensation in the perineum, vulva, and vagina.
- **Menorrhagia** is the medical term for menstrual periods involving abnormally heavy or prolonged bleeding. It is a common concern among premenopausal women.
- **Metrorrhagia** is uterine bleeding at irregular intervals, particularly between the expected menstrual periods.
- **Dysmenorrhea** is painful menstruation, typically involving abdominal cramps.
- In marsupialization of a Bartholin gland, the wound is allowed to heal through **granulation.**
- Endometrial and endocervical specimens should be sent **separately.**
- In all vaginal procedures, the patient's legs are placed in and removed from stirrups **simultaneously.**

Mapping

Here you can see how two common vaginal surgeries map.

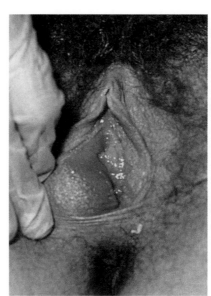

FIG. 7.11 Bartholin abscess. (From Emond RT: *Colour atlas of infectious diseases,* ed 4, St Louis, 2003, Mosby.)

SURGICAL MAPPING
Marsupialization of Bartholin gland

Instruments	Important Anatomy Involved	Pathophysiology
D&C tray	Vaginal mucosa Bartholin gland	Cyst of Bartholin gland

Microbiology/ Wound Classification	Skin Prep/ Incision/Patient position	Pharmacology
Indigenous microorganisms of the vagina Class IV (dirty)	Vaginal prep Elliptical incision Vaginal mucosa Lithotomy position	General anesthesia or local sedation

SURGICAL MAPPING
D&C (dilation & curettage)

Instruments	Important Anatomy Involved	Pathophysiology
D&C tray Telfa for specimen	Cervix Bladder Vagina Uterus	Menorrhagia Metrorrhagia Dysmenorrhea

Microbiology/Wound Classification	Skin Prep/Incision/ Patient position	Pharmacology
Indigenous microorganisms of the vagina Class IV(dirty)	Vaginal prep Lithotomy position	General anesthesia Pudendal block

Use the template available on the Evolve Resources site to map the remaining procedures:
- Hysteroscopy
- Anterior (cystocele) and posterior (rectocele) colporrhaphy
- Labiaplasty
- Vulvectomy

GENITOURINARY SURGERY

Genitorurinary surgeries affect the male reproductive tract (Fig. 7.12) and urinary bladder (Fig. 7.13).
  This section is divided into four parts:
- Endoscopic procedures
- Penile and testicular procedures
- Kidney, ureter, and bladder procedures
- Prostate procedures

Endoscopic Procedures
Procedures
- Cystoscopy
- Cystoscopy TURP (transurethral resection of prostate)
- Cystoscopy TURBT (transurethral resection of bladder tumor)
- Ureteroscopy
- Urethrotomy

Basic Anatomy Involved
- Urethra
- Ureter
- Bladder
- Prostate
- Kidney
- Trigone (triangular region or tissue, in this case the base of the urinary bladder between the openings of the ureters and urethra)

Basic Equipment Required
- Rigid or flexible cystoscope (0-, 30-, and 45-degree lenses)
- Irrigation tubing and pump
- Van Buren sounds
- Ellik evacuator
- Dennis Brown ring retractor
- Cystoscope instruments, obturator, and sheaths, 14F to 30F
- Resectoscope
- Light source
- Camera
- Endoscopic tower
- Imaging system (KUB [kidneys/ureters/bladder] film)
- Ureteral stent
- Urinary ureteral catheters
- Electrocautery
- Laser
- Sorbitol or glycine (non-electrolytic fluid)
- Three-way Foley catheter

Additional Facts to Remember
- The three-way Foley catheter is used in TURP:
  - To induce tamponade
  - To provide:
    - One opening used to inflate the balloon so it remains securely placed
    - One opening to ensure continuous irrigation for adequate flow
    - One opening for continuous drainage to aid monitoring of hemostasis
- Remember to monitor fluid input and output during the procedure.
- The fluid used as distention medium during endoscopic procedures should be non-electrolytic (e.g., sorbitol or glycine), and therefore nonconductive, to permit use with monopolar resectoscopes and prevent electrical burns of the entire bladder.

Mapping
Here are two genitourinary (GU) surgeries:

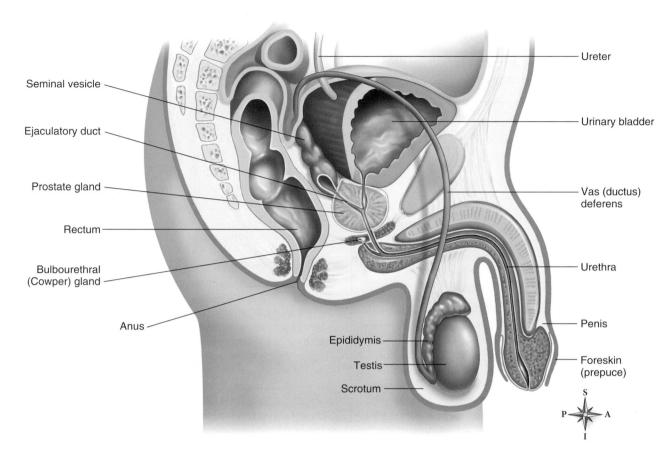

FIG. 7.12 Organization of the male reproductive organs. Sagittal section of pelvis showing placement of male reproductive organs. (From Patton KT, Thibodeau GA: The human body in health & disease, ed 6, St Louis, 2014, Mosby.)

SURGICAL MAPPING

Cystoscopic TURP (transurethral prostatectomy)

Instruments	Important Anatomy Involved	Pathophysiology
Cystoscopy instrumentation: Irrigation, tubing & pump Camera Light source & cable Resectoscope Three-way Foley catheter Ellik evacuator Van Buren sounds Electrocautery	Urethra Prostate Bladder	BPH (benign prostatic hypertrophy)

Microbiology/Wound Classification	Skin Prep/Incision/ Patient position	Pharmacology
Indigenous microorganisms concentrated in the external urethral orifice and navicular fossa, basically consisting of gram-positive aerobic bacteria Class II (clean contaminated)	*Prep:* perineal prep & drape *Position:* lithotomy or low lithotomy *Incision:* none	Spinal/general anesthesia Omniopaque/ Renografin (radiopaque solutions for KUB x-ray series)

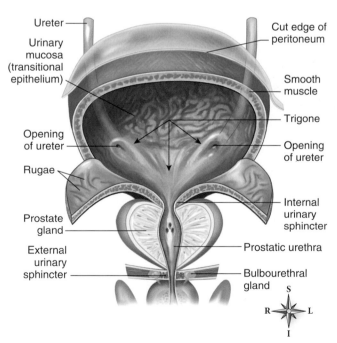

FIG. 7.13 Urinary bladder. Male bladder cut to show the interior. In the male, a large prostate gland surrounds the urethra as it exits from the bladder. (From Patton KT, Thibodeau GA: The human body in health & disease, ed 6, St Louis, 2014, Mosby.)

SURGICAL MAPPING
Ureteroscopy

Instruments	Important Anatomy Involved	Pathophysiology
Ureteroscopy instrumentation irrigation, tubing & Pump Camera Light source & cable Three-way Foley catheter Ureteral stent Van Buren sounds Electrocautery Laser	Urethra Bladder Ureter Kidney	Urinary calculi

Microbiology/Wound Classification	Skin Prep/Incision/ Patient position	Pharmacology
Indigenous microorganisms concentrated in the external urethral orifice and navicular fossa, basically consisting of gram-positive aerobic bacteria Class II (clean contaminated)	*Prep:* perineal prep & drape *Position:* lithotomy	Spinal/general anesthesia Omnipaque/ Renografin (radiopaque solutions for KUB x-ray series)

Go ahead and use the template available on the Evolve Resources site to try mapping the remaining procedures:

- Cystoscopy

- Cystoscopy TURBT (transurethral resection of bladder tumor)
- Urethrotomy

Penile and Testicular Procedures
Procedures

- Hydrocelectomy
- Orchiopexy
- Circumcision (Fig. 7.14)
- Orchiectomy
- Hypospadias and epispadias repair
- Penile prosthesis placement
- Vasvasotomy
- Vasectomy
- Varicocelectomy

Basic Equipment Required

- Genitourinary minor instrument set
- Electrocautery (needle tip)
- Two #15 knife blades

Additional Facts to Remember

- Repair of hypospadias, in which the urethral opening of the penis is on the underside rather than at the tip, may require multiple procedures performed in stages.
- In epispadias, the urethra ends in an opening on the upper aspect (dorsum) of the penis.
- Because of the importance of preserving skin for use as grafts in repair procedures, circumcision is not performed in infants with defects.
- Hypospadias repair also involves the release of chordee to straighten the penis.

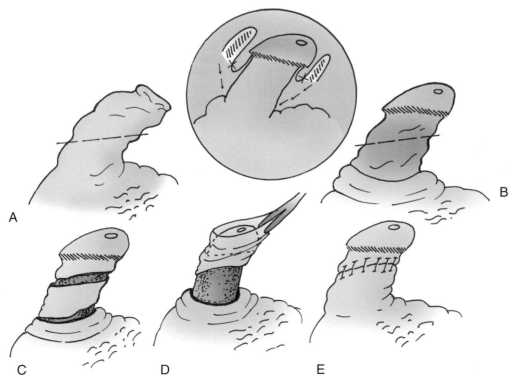

FIG. 7.14 Circumcision. **A,** Initial incision made in the shaft. **B,** Second incision made in subcoronal sulcus. **C,** Amount of tissue to be removed. **D,** Removal of tissue. **E,** Shaft skin sutured to subcoronal skin. (From Holcomb GW, Murphy JP: *Pediatric surgery,* ed 5, Philadelphia, 2010, Saunders.)

- Urethral catheters of 10 to 12 Ch/F for adult women and 10 to 16 Ch/F for adult men are generally chosen; hence, any size smaller than 8F is used for pediatric patients when avoiding damage to the urethra is of major concern.

Mapping

Here's the mapping on two GU procedures that you're likely to encounter in the operating room:

SURGICAL MAPPING

Hypospadias repair

Instruments	Important Anatomy Involved	Pathophysiology
Minor instrument tray	Urethra	Hypospadias
Pediatric Foley catheter	Bladder	

Microbiology/Wound Classification	Skin Prep/Incision/ Patient position	Pharmacology
Indigenous microorganisms concentrated in the external urethral orifice and navicular fossa, basically consisting of gram-positive aerobic bacteria	*Prep:* perineal prep, external genitalia (retracting foreskin as needed) *Incision:* slit-like adjusted Mathieu (SLAM) on dorsal side of penis	Warm normal saline General anesthesia
Class II (clean contaminated)	*Position:* supine	

And now it's your turn; try mapping the remaining procedures, using the template available on the Evolve Resources site:

- Hydrocelectomy
- Orchiopexy
- Circumcision
- Orchiectomy
- Penile prosthesis insertion
- Vasvasotomy
- Vasectomy
- Varicocelectomy

Kidney, Ureter, and Bladder Procedures

See Fig. 7.15 for more information on the urinary system.

Procedures

- Wilms tumor excision
- Nephrectomy (Fig. 7.16)
- Kidney transplant
- Pyelolithotomy
- Cystectomy/ileal conduit procedure
- Marshall-Marchetti-Krantz procedure
- Endoscopic suburethral sling
- Stamey procedure

Basic Laparoscopic Equipment Required

- Light cord
- Camera
- Insufflation or irrigation tubing
- Trocars
- Laparoscopic instruments
- Minor soft instruments
- Fluid to induce distention

Basic Endoscopic Equipment Required

- Light cord
- Camera
- Irrigation tubing
- Trocars
- Cystoscopic instruments

Additional Facts to Remember

- Depending on the surgery, an open or laparoscopic approach may be required.

Endoscopic Procedures

- **Fluid** is used as the medium for **distention**; input and output must be monitored closely so it does not run out.
- **Allen or candy cane stirrups** are used to put the patient in **lithotomy position.**
- The **Stamey procedure** is a retropubic urethropexy approach in which sutures are used to raise the urethra and bladder neck and secure them to the surrounding tissue and bone.

Pyelolithotomy

- If the pleural cavity is to be entered, a chest tube may be necessary, because the 12th rib is removed to permit full visualization of the renal pelvis.
- The left kidney is larger than the right.
- The right kidney is located slightly lower than the left to accommodate the liver.

Ileal Conduit Procedure

- Be prepared for specimens to be taken for frozen sections.
- Seeding must be prevented in the case of tumor excision through isoslation of instruments that have come into contact with cancer cells.
- The patient will have a stoma (ileostomy).

Mapping

Here are a couple of example procedures for you:

SURGICAL MAPPING

Pyelolithotomy

Instruments	Important Anatomy Involved	Pathophysiology
Major laparotomy set	Kidney/area of kidneys	Calculus of the renal pelvis
Abdominal retractors	Ureter	
Vascular tray	Liver, colon, pancreas	
Long instrument tray		
Thoracic tray & chest instruments (available)		

Microbiology/ Wound Classification	Skin Prep/Incision/ Patient position	Pharmacology
Class I (clean)	*Prep:* axilla to midthigh *Position:* lateral with kidney rest (affected side up) *Incision:* flank	General anesthesia

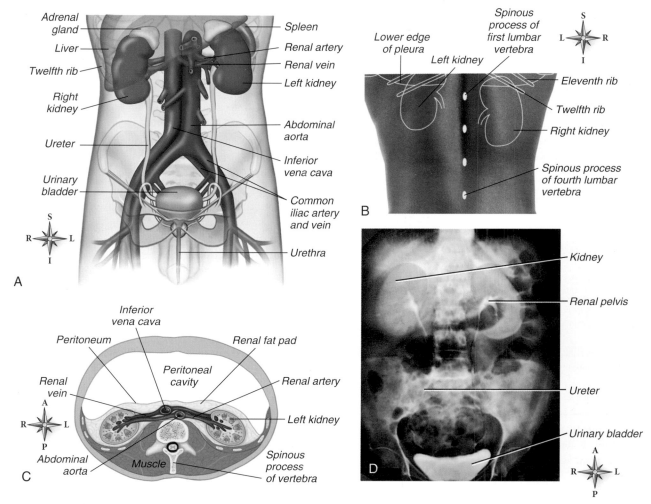

FIG. 7.15 Urinary system. **A,** Anterior view of urinary organs. **B,** Surface markings of the kidneys, 11th and 12th ribs, spinous processes of L1 to L4, and lower edge of pleura viewed from behind. **C,** Horizontal (transverse) section of the abdomen showing the retroperitoneal position of the kidneys. **D,** Colorized x-ray film of the urinary organs. (A, C, D, From Patton KT, Thibodeau GA: The human body in health & disease, ed 6, St Louis, 2014, Mosby. B, From Abrahams P, Hutchings RT, Marks SC: *McMinn's color atlas of human anatomy,* ed 5, St Louis, 2003, Mosby.)

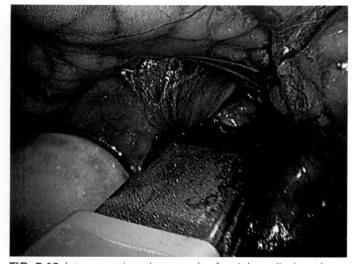

FIG. 7.16 Intraoperative photograph of a right radical nephrectomy. An automatic clip applier is being used to control the renal artery. Note the renal vein to the left of the instrument. (From Becker JM, Stucchi AF: Essentials of surgery, ed 1, Philadelphia, 2006, Saunders.)

SURGICAL MAPPING

Ileal conduit procedure

Instruments	Important Anatomy Involved	Pathophysiology
Major laparotomy tray	Bladder	Malignancy of the
Intestinal tray	Prostate	bladder and
Bookwalter retractor	Ileum	nearby tissues
Stapling devices for bowel	Kidneys	
Vascular tray	Ureters	
Stoma bag		
Ureteral stents		

Microbiology/ Wound Classification	Skin Prep/Incision/ Patient position	Pharmacology
Class IV	*Prep:* midchest to both thighs	General anesthesia
	Incision: midline vertical abdominal	
	Position: supine with laparotomy draping	

Try mapping the remaining procedures using the template available on the Evolve Resources site:

- Wilms tumor excision
- Nephrectomy
- Kidney transplant
- Marshall-Marchetti-Krantz procedure
- Endoscopic suburethral sling
- Stamey procedure

Prostate Procedures

These surgeries may be performed endoscopically (laparoscopically) or as open procedures.

Procedures

- Prostatectomy (Fig. 7.17)
- Suprapubic prostatectomy
- Laparoscopic robot-assisted prostatectomy
- Implantation of radioactive seeds into the prostate

Basic Laparoscopic Equipment Required

- Light cord
- Camera
- Insufflation tubing
- Trocars
- Laparoscopic instruments
- Minor soft Instruments

Additional Facts to Remember

- In endoscopic procedures, fluid is used as the medium for distention.
- Allen or candy cane stirrups are used to place the patient in the lithotomy position.
- A Foley catheter is inserted and maintained on the sterile field.

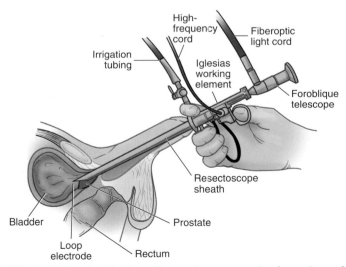

FIG. 7.17 Sectional view illustrating removal of portion of hypertrophied middle lobe of prostate gland with Iglesias resectoscope. (From Rothrock JC: Alexander's care of the patient in surgery, ed 15, St Louis, 2015, Mosby.)

Mapping

Here's how one of these procedures looks when mapped:

SURGICAL MAPPING

Suprapubic prostatectomy

Instruments	Important Anatomy Involved	Pathophysiology
Major laparotomy set	Ureter	Prostate cancer
Abdominal retractors (Judd-Mason)	Bladder	
GU instrument tray	Urethra	
Long instrument tray	Prostate	
Electrocautery		
Hemoclips		
Suprapubic & Foley catheters		

Microbiology/ Wound Classification	Skin Prep/Incision/ Patient position	Pharmacology
Class II (clean contaminated)	*Prep:* axillae to midthigh, perineal prep; laparotomy draping in combination with perineal draping of scrotum	General anesthesia
	Incision: low transverse	
	Position: supine/frog leg shoulder brace for Trendelenburg rotation	

The remaining procedures are yours to map!

- Prostatectomy
- Laparoscopic robot-assisted prostatectomy
- Implantation of radioactive seeds into the prostate

ORTHOPEDIC SURGERIES

Orthopedic surgeries involve the musculoskeletal system (Fig. 7.18).

- Arthroscopic procedures
- Open reduction/internal fixation (ORIF) and amputation procedures
- Arthroplasty procedures
- Open shoulder procedures and tendon repair

Arthroscopic Procedures
Procedures

- Arthroscopy of the knee (diagnostic)
- Arthroscopy of the knee (anterior cruciate ligament [ACL] reconstruction)
- Arthroscopy of the shoulder (diagnostic)
- Arthroscopy of the shoulder (Bankart procedure)

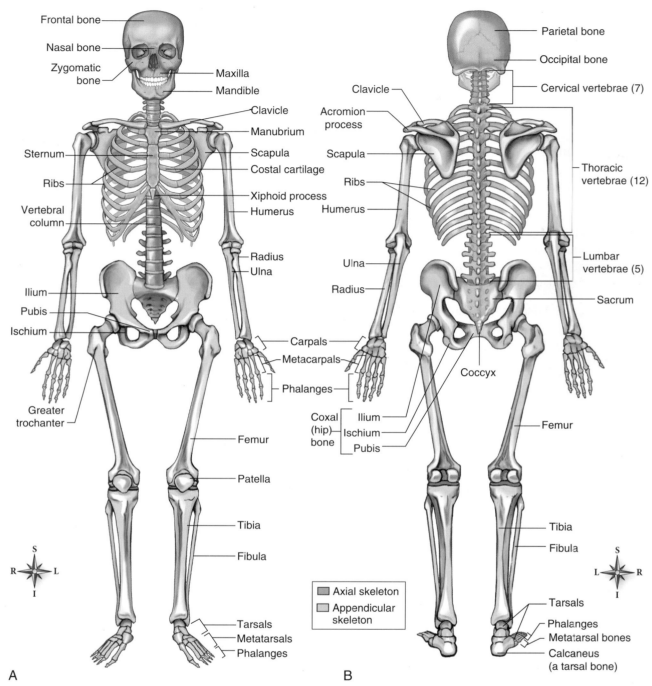

FIG. 7.18 Human skeleton. The axial skeleton is distinguished by a blue tint. **A,** Anterior view. **B,** Posterior view. (From Patton KT, Thibodeau GA: The human body in health & disease, ed 6, St Louis, 2014, Mosby.)

- Arthroscopy of the shoulder (acromioplasty)
- Arthroscopy of the hip
- Arthroscopy of the ankle

Basic Equipment for Arthroscopic Procedures

- Basic orthopedic instrument tray
- Irrigation tubing and pump
- Arthroscopic tower

- Tourniquet
- Arthroscopic instrument tray
- Arthroscope with 30- and 70-degree lenses
- Arthroscopic shaver
- Camera
- Light source and cord
- 3000-mL bags of fluid (distention medium)
- Power drill and saw

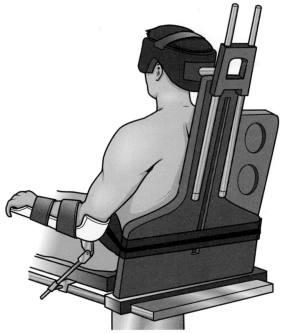

FIG. 7.19 Beach chair–style shoulder positioner allows distraction of the joint for visualization. (From Rothrock JC, Alexander SM: Alexander's surgical procedures, ed 1, St. Louis, 2012, Mosby.)

- Suture anchors
- Beach chair positioner (for shoulder procedures; Fig. 7.19)

Additional Facts to Remember

- The patient is placed in the supine position/modified "beach chair" (Fowler) position for shoulder surgeries.
- For knee operations, the patient is placed in the supine/lateral position with the knee to be operated on placed below the break of the table.
- Before any arthroscopic procedure, you must check all videoscopic equipment, prime the pump, and white-balance the scope.
- Remember to monitor fluid input and output during procedure.
- Remember to monitor tourniquet time carefully:
  - The surgeon should be informed once the cuff has been inflated for the first 60 minutes.
  - The recommended inflation time for the arms is 60 minutes; it is 90 minutes for the legs.
  - When the recommended time limit has been reached, the cuff should be deflated for 15 minutes to permit reperfusion of the extremity, after which the cuff may be reinflated for another recommended time period (i.e., 60 or 90 minutes).
  - The limb should be re-exsanguinated before reinflation to help prevent the formation of venous thromboses.

Mapping

Here's the map of one extremely common arthroscopic procedure:

SURGICAL MAPPING

Arthroscopic ACL reconstruction

Instruments	Important Anatomy Involved	Pathophysiology
Arthroscopy instrumentation: arthroscope, irrigation, tubing, pump	Knee Femur Tibial plateau	MRI findings (i.e., torn ACL)
Camera	Meniscus	
Light source and cord	ACL	
Arthroscopic tower	PCL	
Fixation device, bone plugs, screws	MCL	
Power drill and saw		
Arthroscopic shaver		
Tourniquet		

Microbiology/ Wound Classification	Skin Prep/Incision/ Patient position	Pharmacology
No indigenous micro-organisms in these structures Clean class I	*Prep:* entire leg circumferentially, from toes to groin; Extremity draping with impervious stockinette *Incision:* 2 stab incisions on medial & lateral knee joint capsule; vertical incision over patellar tendon (if harvesting graft from patient) *Position:* supine with padded lateral post; affected knee joint extended over break of table	General anesthesia, epidural, or spinal block

Now it's your turn: Use the template on the Evolve Resources site to try your hand at mapping the remaining procedures:

- Arthroscopy of the knee (diagnostic)
- Arthroscopy of the shoulder (diagnostic)
- Arthroscopy of the shoulder (Bankart procedure)
- Arthroscopy of the shoulder (acromioplasty)
- Arthroscopy of the hip
- Arthroscopy of the ankle

OPEN REDUCTION/INTERNAL FIXATION AND AMPUTATION PROCEDURES

In this section, we'll cover a range of orthopedic surgeries, many involving open reduction/internal fixation (ORIF).

Procedures

- AKA (above-the-knee amputation)
- BKA (below-the-knee amputation)
- ORIF of radius (Fig. 7.20)
- External fixation of Colles fracture
- ORIF of hip fracture
- ORIF of humerus
- ORIF of femur (femoral nail/femoral rodding)

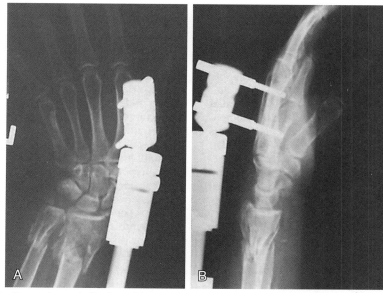

FIG. 7.20 A, Comminuted displaced intraarticular distal radius fracture (a.k.a. Colle fracture). B, After open reduction and internal fixation (ORIF) surgery with anatomic alignment. (From Donatelli RA, Wooden MJ: Orthopaedic physical therapy, ed 4, St Louis, 2010, Churchill Livingstone.)

- Bunionectomy (Keller, Austin)
- Triple arthrodesis
- ORIF of tibia
- ORIF of fibula

Basic Anatomy Affected

- All short and long bones
- Cancellous and cortical bone

Basic Equipment Required

- Fracture table
- Special arm board
- Imaging equipment: fluoroscopy, C-arm, image intensifier
- Power equipment: drill, saw, reamer
- Tourniquet (Esmarch)
- Minor and major orthopedic instrument sets
- Fixation implants: screws, plates, prosthesis
- Draping: extremity drape, split sheet, stockinette as needed
- Polymethylmethacrylate bone cement
- Scavenging system
- Screws: cancellous, cortical, cannulated
- Gigli saw
- Spacesuit/hood

Additional Facts to Remember

- Remember to verify that the correct implants are available and have been supplied **before** the patient is brought into the surgical suite.
  Monitor tourniquet time carefully.
  Most screws are self-tapping, but it's important to remember the sequence of steps in screw insertion nonetheless:

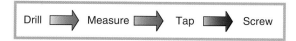

- Know the various types of fractures (Fig. 7.21)

Mapping

Here's the map for one common orthopedic surgery.

SURGICAL MAPPING

ORIF of hip fracture

Instruments	Important Anatomy Involved	Pathophysiology
Major orthopedic tray	Pelvis	Hip fracture
Power equipment (drill, reamer)	Hip joint	
	Femur	
Cannulated screw or DHS (dynamic hip compression) tray	Femoral head	
	Femoral neck	
	Trochanter	
Pulse lavage	Acetabulum	
	C-arm	

Microbiology/ Wound Classification	Skin Prep/Incision/ Patient position	Pharmacology
Class I (clean)	*Prep:* beginning at hip joint, midline of abdomen on operative side up to midchest as far laterally as possible, and entire operative leg	Warm normal saline
		General anesthesia
	Incision: from greater trochanter to implant site on affected leg	
	Draping: 4 towels; incise drape and laparotomy sheet	
	Position: supine on fracture table.	

Ready to map? Here are the remaining procedures:

- AKA (above-the-knee amputation)
- BKA (below-the-knee amputation)
- ORIF of radius
- External fixation of Colles fracture
- ORIF of humerus
- ORIF of femur (femoral nail)

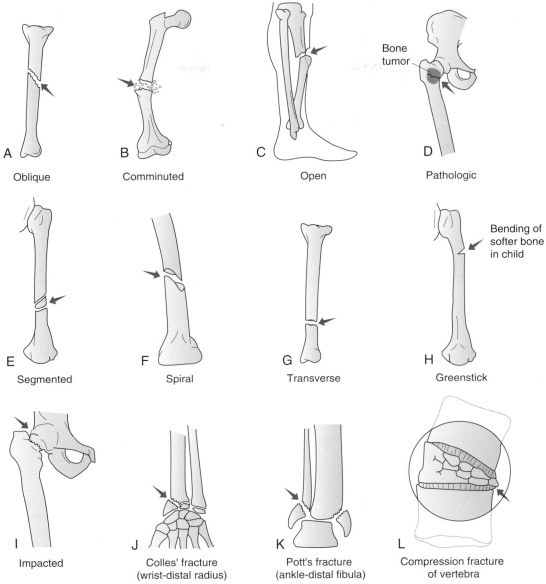

FIG. 7.21 Types of fractures. (From VanMeter KC, Hubert RJ: Gould's pathophysiology for the health professions, ed 5, St Louis, 2014, Saunders.)

- Bunionectomy (Keller, Austin)
- Triple arthrodesis
- ORIF of tibia
- ORIF of fibula

Arthroplasty Procedures
Procedures
- Total knee arthroplasty
- Total hip arthroplasty
- Total shoulder arthroplasty
- Total ankle joint arthroplasty
- Metacarpal arthroplasty

Basic Arthroplasty Equipment Required
- Power equipment (Fig. 7.22)
- Polymethylmethacrylate (PMMA; bone cement)
- Cement-mixing system

- Implants
- Major orthopedic tray
- Tourniquets for knee and ankle
- Implant trays
- Spacesuits or hood systems
- Pulse lavage
- Cement gun
- Beach chair positioner (shoulder procedures)

Additional Facts to Remember
- Cement mixing must be timed.
- Check the batteries in your power equipment before each procedure to ensure full charges.
- Pulse lavage is used before cement application to prevent embolus formation.
- An abduction pillow is applied immediately after the procedure to help prevent dislocation.

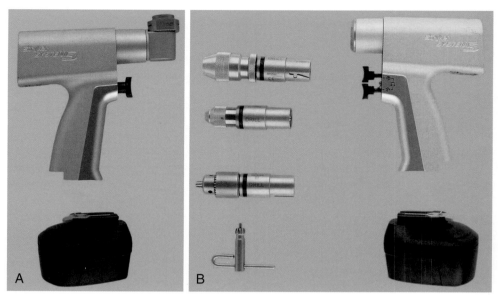

FIG. 7.22 Pneumatic-powered surgical instruments for large bone procedures. **A,** Oscillating saw and battery. **B,** Dual-trigger rotary handpiece with attachments and battery. From Tighe SM: *Instrumentation for the operating room: a photographic manual,* ed 9, St Louis, 2016, Mosby.

Mapping

Here's one common arthroplastic procedure all mapped out:

SURGICAL MAPPING

Total hip arthroplasty

Instruments	Important Anatomy Involved	Pathophysiology
Major orthopedic tray	Pelvis	Osteoarthritis of
Power equipment (drill, reamer)	Hip joint	the hip
	Femur	
Implants	Femoral head	
Implant trays	Femoral neck	
PMMA	Trochanter	
Cement-mixing system	Acetabulum	
Abduction pillow		
Beanbag		
Pulse lavage		

Microbiology/ Wound Classification	Skin Prep/Incision/ Patient position	Pharmacology
Class I (clean)	*Prep:* beginning around hip, midline of abdomen on operative side up to midchest as far laterally as possible, and entire operative leg & foot	General anesthesia
	Draping: 4 towels, incision drape, U drape, split sheet, stockinette, Coban	
	Position: lateral with bean-bag (affected side up)	
	Incision: posterolateral, centered over greater trochanter	

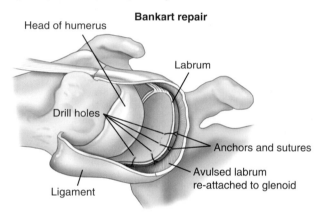

Bankart repair

Head of humerus

Labrum

Drill holes

Anchors and sutures

Avulsed labrum re-attached to glenoid

Ligament

The labrum is re-attached to the glenoid using surgical anchors and sutures.

FIG. 7.23 Bankart procedure to restore stability of shoulder.

OK, your turn! Map the remaining procedures, using the template on the Evolve Resources site:

- Total knee arthroplasty
- Total shoulder arthroplasty
- Total ankle joint arthroplasty
- Metacarpal arthroplasty

Open Shoulder and Tendon Repair Procedures

Procedures

- Bankart procedure (Fig. 7.23)
- Bristow procedure
- Open rotator cuff repair
- Putti-Platt reconstruction
- Achilles tendon repair

Basic Equipment Required for Open Shoulder Procedures

- Major orthopedic tray
- Power equipment: drill ,saw, reamer
- Suture anchors
- Shoulder immobilizer
- Beach chair positioner

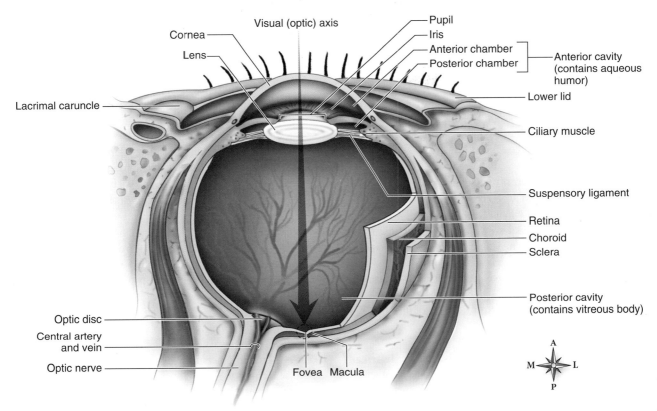

FIG. 7.24 Horizontal section through the left eyeball. The eye as viewed from above. (From Patton KT, Thibodeau GA: The human body in health & disease, ed 6, St Louis, 2014, Mosby.)

Basic Equipment Required for Achilles Tendon Repair

- Minor orthopedic tray
- Tendon graspers
- Tendon strippers
- Tourniquet

Additional Facts to Remember

- Shoulder procedures require the patient to be in the supine/semi-Fowler/beach chair position.
- Patients undergoing Achilles tendon surgery are placed in the prone position.
- Other tendon procedures require the supine position or some other position, depending on the surgeon's preference.
- The patient will be placed in a splint or cast immediately after Achilles tendon repair.

Mapping

Here you can see how one important tendon surgery is performed.

SURGICAL MAPPING

Achilles tendon repair

Instruments	Important Anatomy Involved	Pathophysiology
Major orthopedic tray	Calcaneus	Tendon rupture
Drill	Gastrocnemius muscle	
Ethibond nonabsorbable suture for Krackow stitch repair		

Microbiology/ Wound Classification	Skin Prep/Incision/ Patient position	Pharmacology
Class I (clean)	*Prep:* starting at ankle joint and extending up to midthigh tourniquet circumferentially	General anesthesia or spinal block
	Extremity draping, stockinette	
	Incision: posteromedial incision 1 cm medial to tendon.	
	Position: prone	

Go ahead and try to map these orthopedic surgeries, using the template on the Evolve Resources site. Ready?

- Bankart procedure
- Bristow procedure
- Open rotator cuff repair
- Putti-Platt reconstruction

OPHTHALMIC SURGERIES

Let's go over the most common surgeries of the eye (Fig. 7.24).

Procedures

- Strabismus correction
- Scleral buckle
- Keratoplasty

- Cataract removal
- Vitrectomy

Facts to Remember
Cataract Procedures

- Two types:
  - **Intracapsular** cataract extraction (Fig. 7.25)
    - This surgery involves a larger incision at the corneo-scleral junction or corneal margin.
    - **Suturing** is involved to close the incision
    - The entire capsule is **removed**
    - Lens is replaced with an **IOL (intraocular lens)**
  - **Extracapsular** cataract extraction
    - This surgery involves a **small incision** at the corneo-scleral junction or corneal margin, followed by **iridotomy** (an incision into the iris).
    - Because the incision is self-sealing, usually **no suturing** is required.
    - The lens is **replaced** with an IOL (intraocular lens).
- Drugs used in cataract surgery:
  - **Balanced salt solution (BSS)**
  - **Healon** (sodium hyaluronate): This viscoelastic **lubricant** maintains separation between the tissues to protect the endothelium and keep the deep anterior chamber from collapsing, permitting efficient manipulation and less trauma to the corneal endothelium and surrounding tissues.
- The cornea **protects** the eye, **allows light** into the eye, and **bends light rays** onto the lens, which in turn focuses the light on the retina.
- Only the **central part** of the cornea is replaced in cornea transplantation.
- A **trephine** is an instrument used to make a cut around the cornea and into the anterior chamber.

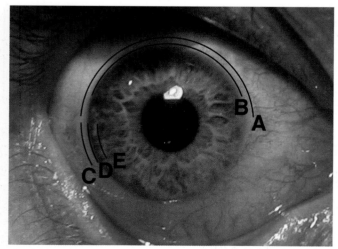

FIG. 7.25 External entry site for standard cataract incisions. A, Superior intracapsular incision. B, Superior extracapsular incision. C, Temporal scleral (phacoemulsification) incision. D, Temporal limbal (phacoemulsification) incision. E, Temporal clear corneal (phacoemulsification) incision. (From Bruce A, Loughnan M: Anterior eye disease and therapeutics A-Z, ed 2, Sydney, 2011, Churchill Livingstone.)

Strabismus Repair

- The procedure is performed to change the **alignment** of the eyes, either by loosening or tightening the rectus muscles.
- Misalignments take three forms:
  - In **esotropia**, one or both eyes turn inward.
  - In **exotropia** (a.k.a. divergent squint or walleye), the eyes are deviated outward.
  - **Amblyopia** is impaired or dim vision that is not the result of an obvious defect or change in the eye.
- Recession: **reattachment** of the medial rectus muscle farther back on the eye
- Resection: **surgical shortening** of the lateral rectus muscle

Scleral Buckle

- This procedure (Fig. 7.26) involves the **placement of a piece of silicone** (a semi-hard plastic) around the sclera (white part of the eye), pushing the sclera toward the middle of the eye and replacing a detached retina to its original state.
- The buckle remains in the eye **indefinitely** unless infection develops after surgery.
- Cryopexy or laser photocoagulation is used to **create a scar** to seal the tear in the retina.
- Sometimes **vitrectomy** (see below) is performed in conjuction with the scleral buckle procedure.

Vitrectomy

- An incision is made through the **pars plana layer,** one of the three layers of the eye near the point where iris and sclera join.
- The main purpose of the vitreous humor, the gel found in the posterior chamber, is to **maintain sufficient pressure** in the eye to keep the eyeball from collapsing.
- The instrument used to cut and aspirate the vitreous humor is called an **ocutome.**
- Intraocular **gases**, mixed with sterile air, are used to flattened the detached retina and keep it attached while healing takes place:
  - **Sulfur hexafluoride** (SF_6)
  - **Per-fluoro-ethane** (C_2F_6)
  - **Per-fluoro-propane** (C_3F_8)
- **Silicone oil** may also be used to keep the retina attached after surgery.

Drugs Used in Ophthalmic Surgery

- **Atropine** is a cycloplegic (paralyzes accommodation and inhibits focusing).
- **Phenylephrine** (2.5% or 10%) is a mydriatric (dilates the pupil and permits focusing).
- **Acetylcholine chloride 1%** is a miotic (causes the pupil to constrict).
- **BSS** (discussed above) is an irrigation solution.
- **Mannitol** is a hyperosmotic agent (reduces intraocular pressure).
- **Tetracaine hydrochloride** is a topical anesthetic agent.
- **Dexamethasone** is a corticosteroid used for its antiinflammatory effects

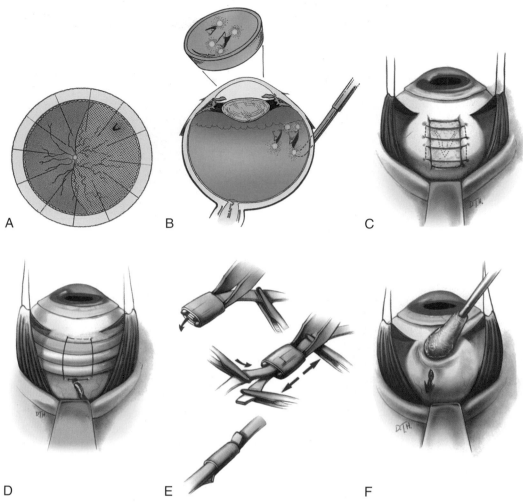

FIG. 7.26 Scleral buckling operation for treatment of retinal detachment. **A,** Diagram of retina showing detachment of retina of temporal half of left eye, with retinal tear at equator of globe at 1:30 clock position. **B,** Examination of fundus with the use of an ophthalmoscope and handheld lens and depression of sclera with a diathermy electrode. Surgeon visualizes field and places electrode beneath retinal tear; burn mark is made on sclera at site of retinal tear with diathermy electrode. **C,** A sponge is sutured in place over treated site of retinal tear. **D,** Band and tire are used to encircle the eye. **E,** Placement of Watzke silicone sleeve is one method of securing edges of encircling band. **F,** Small incision is made through sclera, and choroid is finely incised to allow subretinal fluid to drain. (From Ryan SJ et al: *Retina,* vol 3, ed 4, St Louis, 2006, Mosby.)

Mapping

Let's see how the procedures we've just discussed look when they're mapped.

SURGICAL MAPPING

Strabismus correction

Instruments	Important Anatomy Involved	Pathophysiology
Ophthalmic tray	6 Extrinsic muscles: Superior rectus Inferior rectus Medial rectus, Lateral rectus, Superior oblique Inferior oblique	Esotropia Exotropia Amblyopia

Microbiology/ Wound Classification	Skin Prep/Incision/ Patient position	Pharmacology
No indigenous microorganisms Class I (clean)	*Prep:* eyelid and margins, inner and outer canthus, brows, and face, ending at the chin	Retrobulbar or peribulbar block; sometimes general anesthesia

Your turn! Go ahead and try mapping the remaining procedures in the template available on the Evolve Resources site:

- Vitrectomy
- Scleral buckle

SURGICAL MAPPING

Extracapsular cataract removal

Instruments	Important Anatomy Involved	Pathophysiology
Cataract ophthalmic tray	Lens	Aging
Phaco machine	Ciliary process	Traumatic injury
	Iris	Harmful chemical
	Suspensory ligament	exposure
	Pupil	Congenital cataract

Microbiology/ Wound Classification	Skin Prep/Incision/ Patient position	Pharmacology
No indigenous microorganisms	*Prep:* eyelid and margins, inner and outer canthus, brows, and face ending at the chin	Retrobulbar block with conscious sedation
Class I (clean)	*Incision:* corneoscleral or corneal	
	Position: supine	

SURGICAL MAPPING

Keratoplasty

Instruments	Important Anatomy Involved	Pathophysiology
Ophthalmic tray	Sclera	Corneal scarring
Trephine or Cottingham punch	Cornea	Severe fungal, viral, or bacterial infection
		Corneal dystrophy

Microbiology/ Wound Classification	Skin Prep/Incision/ Patient position	Pharmacology
No indigenous microorganisms	*Prep:* Eyelid and margins, inner and outer canthus, brows, face ending at chin	General anesthesia
Class I (clean)	*Incision:* around cornea and into anterior chamber	Tetracaine drops after induction of general anesthesia
	Position: supine	

ORAL AND MAXILLOFACIAL SURGERY

Procedures

- Le Fort I osteotomy (see Fig. 7.27 for details of the Le Fort procedures that you'll need to know)
- Le Fort II osteotomy
- Le Fort III osteotomy
- Orbital floor fracture repair
- Tooth extraction/odontectomy

Facts to Remember

LeFort I Osteotomy

- Performed when lower maxillary deficiency is accompanied by inadequate zygomatic projection and the orbit is not involved
- Incision: gingivobuccal sulcus
- Wound classification: class II (clean contaminated), because the incision is made in the transoral vestibule

LeFort II and II Osteotomies

- LeFort II and III are performed as part of major treatment plan in craniofacial dysotosis syndrome, also known as Crouzon

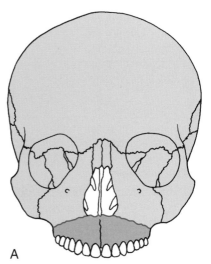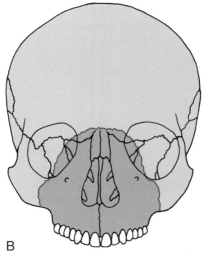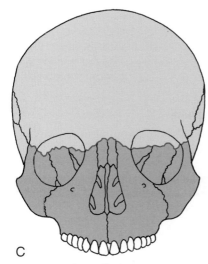

FIG. 7.27 Le Fort midfacial fractures. A, Le Fort I fracture separating inferior portion of maxilla in horizontal fashion, extending from piriform aperture of nose to pterygoid maxillary suture area. B, Le Fort II fracture involving separation of maxilla and nasal complex from cranial base, zygomatic orbital rim area, and pterygoid maxillary suture area. C, Le Fort III fracture (i.e., craniofacial separation), which is a complete separation of midface at level of naso-orbital-ethmoid complex and zygomaticofrontal suture area. The fracture also extends through orbits bilaterally. (From Hupp JR, Ellis E III, Tucker MR: Contemporary oral and maxillofacial surgery, ed 6, St Louis, 2014, Mosby.)

syndrome, a rare genetic disorder that may be evident at birth (congenital) or become apparent during infancy. The disorder is characterized by distinctive craniofacial malformations.

- Diagnosis of facial fractures is made with the use of x-ray and CT scan.
- For repair of any facial fracture, **Triclosan** (broad-spectrum antimicrobial agent) and **PCMX** (parachlorometaxylenol) are used as prep, but these solutions should not be allowed to enter the patient's eyes. Warm sterile water is used for rinsing.

- **Hexachlorophene** and **chlorhexidine** are not used on the face because they are ototoxic. A sterile cotton ball should be placed in the ear during prep of the surgical site.

Maxillomandibular Fixation (MMF)

- This the name given to the application of **arch bars** (Fig. 7.28).
- If this procedure performed for Le Fort I, II, or III, the surgical technologist in the scrub role must have two setups ready.
- Wire, 24- or 26-gauge, is used to close the jaw.

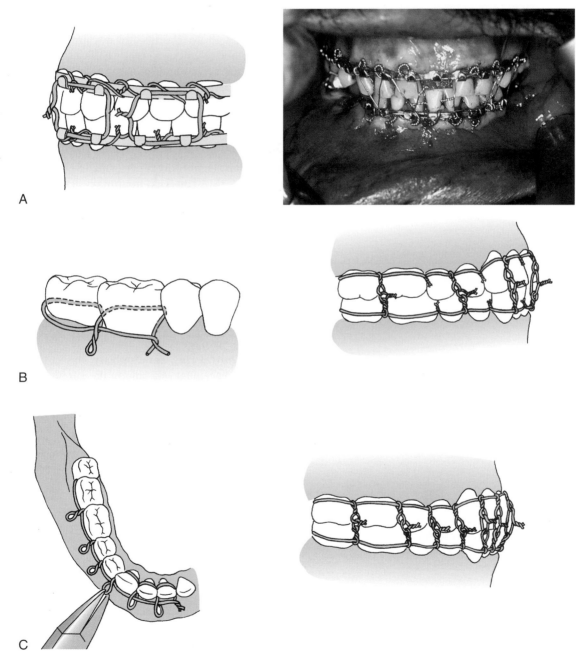

FIG. 7.28 Intermaxillary fixation wiring techniques. **A,** Arch bar intermaxillary fixation. **B,** Ivy loop wiring technique. **C,** Continuous loop wiring technique. (From Hupp JR, Ellis E III, Tucker MR: Contemporary oral and maxillofacial surgery, ed 6, St Louis, 2014, Mosby; modified from Kruger E, Schilli W: Oral and maxillofacial traumatology, vol 1, Chicago, IL, 1982, Quintessence.)

- Wire cutters are kept with the patient **at all times** after surgery and discharge to permit immediate access to the mouth in case of airway emergency.
- These procedures are categorized as class IV (dirty) because of their location in the mouth.

Mapping

Here's the mapping for one of the LeFort procedures.

SURGICAL MAPPING

LeFort II (pyramidal maxillary fracture)

Instruments	Important Anatomy Involved	Pathophysiology
Dental instruments Internal fixation system	Ethmoid, frontal, maxillary, zygomatic bones Vomer Infraorbital nerve Nasolacrimal duct	Blunt trauma Motor vehicle crash

Microbiology/ Wound Classification	Skin Prep/Incision/ Patient position	Pharmacology
No indigenous microorganisms in area of incision Class I (clean)	*Prep:* entire face, from hairline to sternal notch *Incision:* mucogingival *Position:* supine	General anesthesia

Go ahead and try mapping the remaining oral and maxillofacial procedures on your own, using the template available on the Evolve Resources site:

- Le Fort I osteotomy
- Le Fort III osteotomy
- Orbital floor fracture repair
- Tooth extraction/odontectomy

CARDIOTHORACIC SURGERY

The heart (Fig. 7.29) is the subject of a wide range of surgical repairs.

Procedures

- CABG (coronary artery bypass graft)
- Intraaortic balloon pump insertion
- Ventricular assist device (VAD) insertion
- Valve replacement: aortic, mitral, tricuspid
- Orthotopic heart transplant
- Thoracotomy
- Thoracoscopy/VATS (video-assisted thoracoscopy)
- Mediastinoscopy
- Bronchoscopy

Facts to Remember

- Be sure that you've memorized the **cardiac cycle** (Fig. 7.30) and **heart conduction system** (Fig. 7.31).

Heart-Lung Machine

- This apparatus (see Fig. 7.32 for a detailed explanation of how it works) is used to **shunt blood** from the heart. A venous cannula is inserted inside the superior inferior venae cavae for deoxygenated blood. Sometimes the cannula is inserted into right atrium if the aortic pressure is high.
- The cannula used in **two-stage (bicaval)** venous cannulation has holes in the distal ends. *Bicaval* means that both cavae are cannulated. A two-stage cannula is inserted into the inferior vena cava (IVC) through the right atrial appendage. The cannula has distal holes that pick up blood from the IVC; the proximal holes pick up blood from the superior vena cava (SVC) and right atrium.
- When an arterial cannula is placed in the aortic artery, the surgeon always **clamps and unclamps** the cannula to allow the blood to enter and remove the air.
- Femoral artery and vein cannulation is performed when **partial bypass** is needed to support the patient's circulation in surgical resection of the descending thoracic aorta and ascending aorta.

Off-Pump Coronary Artery Bypass (OPCAB)

- **Median sternotomy** is performed to provide access.
- The left IMA (**internal mammary artery**) is harvested.

Valve Repair and Replacement

- A **heart-lung machine** is required.
- Mitral valve repair (left heart) is performed in one of two ways:
  - **Mitral commissurotomy** is the opening of the commissure that brings the cups of the valve together. This technique is used to relieve stenosis when the valve leaflets are sufficiently flexible to allow it. A Gerbode or Tubbs dilator is used to break them apart.
  - In **mitral ring annuloplasty**, the valve is repaired with the placement of a ring in the annulus to allow the valve leaflets to come together more efficiently.
- Similar procedures are performed in **tricuspid valve repair.**

CABG (Coronary Artery Bypass Graft)

- The saphenous vein or internal mammary artery (IMA) is used.

Heart Transplantation

Heart transplantation (Fig. 7.33) may be performed in one of two ways:

Orthotopic

- This procedure, involving replacement of one heart with another, is the more commonly performed of the two methods.
- It involves end-to-end anastomosis of the superior vena cava and inferior vena cava, as well as anastomosis of the left atrium, pulmonary artery, and aorta to the recipient.

Heterotopic

- In this procedure, also known as "piggyback" transplantation, a donor heart is inserted into a recipient's right pleural

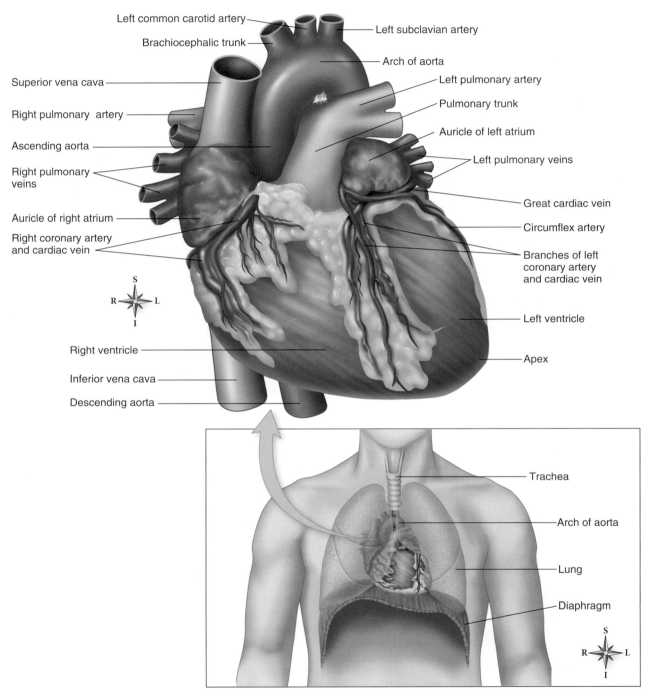

FIG. 7.29 The heart. The heart and major blood vessels viewed from the front (anterior). Inset shows the relationship of the heart to other structures in the thoracic cavity. (From Patton KT, Thibodeau GA: The human body in health & disease, ed 6, St Louis, 2014, Mosby.)

THE CARDIAC CYCLE

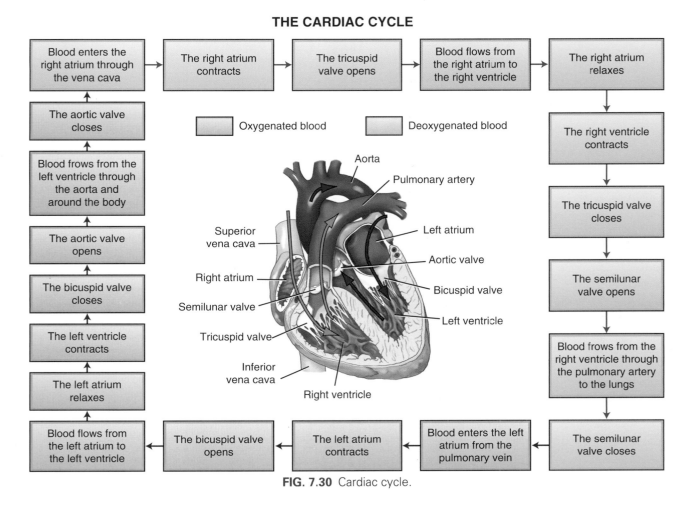

Blood enters the right atrium through the vena cava → The right atrium contracts → The tricuspid valve opens → Blood flows from the right atrium to the right ventricle → The right atrium relaxes

The aortic valve closes ↑

☐ Oxygenated blood   ☐ Deoxygenated blood

The right ventricle contracts ↓

Blood frows from the left ventricle through the aorta and around the body ↑

The tricuspid valve closes ↓

The aortic valve opens ↑

The semilunar valve opens ↓

The bicuspid valve closes ↑

The left ventricle contracts ↑

Blood frows from the right ventricle through the pulmonary artery to the lungs ↓

The left atrium relaxes ↑

Blood flows from the left atrium to the left ventricle ← The bicuspid valve opens ← The left atrium contracts ← Blood enters the left atrium from the pulmonary vein ← The semilunar valve closes

Labels on heart diagram: Aorta, Pulmonary artery, Superior vena cava, Left atrium, Aortic valve, Right atrium, Bicuspid valve, Semilunar valve, Left ventricle, Tricuspid valve, Inferior vena cava, Right ventricle

FIG. 7.30 Cardiac cycle.

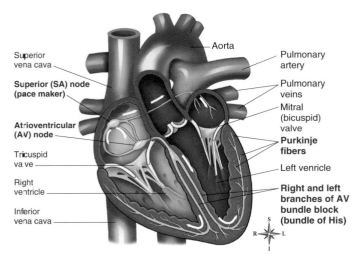

FIG. 7.31 Conduction system of the heart. Specialized cardiac muscle cells *(yellow)* in the wall of the heart rapidly conduct an electrical impulse throughout the myocardium. The signal is initiated by the sinoatrial *(SA)* node (pacemaker) and spreads to the rest of the atrial myocardium and to the atrioventricular *(AV)* node. The AV node then initiates a signal that is conducted through the ventricular myocardium by way of the AV bundle (of His) and Purkinje fibers. Labels for parts of the heart's conduction system are highlighted in red. (From Patton KT, Thibodeau GA: The human body in health & disease, ed 6, St Louis, 2014, Mosby.)

Labels on Fig 7.31: Superior vena cava, Superior (SA) node (pace maker), Atrioventricular (AV) node, Tricuspid valve, Right ventricle, Inferior vena cava, Aorta, Pulmonary artery, Pulmonary veins, Mitral (bicuspid) valve, Purkinje fibers, Left ventricle, Right and left branches of AV bundle block (bundle of His)

cavity, allowing the donor heart to work in tandem with the recipient's own.

- This surgery is usually chosen when a significant disparity in size exists between a donor's small heart and a recipient's large one.

Bronchoscopy

- This invasive procedure is used for the diagnosis, evaluation, and treatment of various conditions. Examples include:
  - Retrieval of foreign objects from the bronchus in pediatric patients
  - Laser guidance in the treatment of endobronchial tumors
  - Postoperative evaluation of transplanted lungs
- Because the bronchoscope is inserted through the mouth but there is no wound, the procedure is categorized in wound classification V (unclassified).
- Foreign bodies lodge more easily in the right bronchus because it's wider and straighter than the left one.
- A rigid bronchoscope is employed in pediatric patients to remove foreign bodies. This instrument, with its larger diameter and hollow working channel, can be used in ways that the pediatric flexible bronchoscope cannot:
  - It facilitates the passage of various grasping devices and other instruments.
  - It permits suctioning of clotted blood, foreign bodies, and thick secretions.

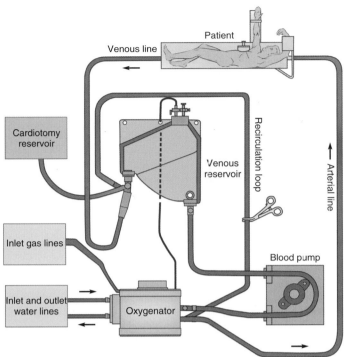

FIG. 7.32 Cardiopulmonary bypass circuit. Venous blood is drained by gravity from the right atrium or venae cavae into an oxygenator that incorporates a blood reservoir and a heat exchanger, which warms or cools the blood as needed. The ventilating gas flowing into the oxygenator removes carbon dioxide and adds oxygen to the blood. Saturated blood leaves the oxygenator and is pumped from the reservoir into the arterial system by the use of a roller pump. Filters and monitors are incorporated into the circuit. Additional roller pumps are used to suction shed blood from the pericardial well and the intracardiac chambers (cardiotomy suckers); the blood is returned to the cardiotomy reservoir. Another roller pump is used to vent air and blood through a right superior pulmonary venous catheter that is inserted into the left ventricle. (From Buxton B et al: *Ischemic heart disease surgical management,* London, 1999, Mosby.)

Mediastinoscopy

- This procedure is performed to aid evaluation of lymph node involvement or mediastinal tumors in patients with lung cancer.
- Lesions commonly found include:
  - Neurogenic tumor (in children)
  - Thymoma, lymphoma (in adults)
- An incision is made at the suprasternal notch.
- The wound is categorized as class I (clean).

Thoracoscopy and Thoracotomy

- In thoracoscopy, the thorax **cannot be expanded** through insufflation because it is constricted by the ribcage.
- In both procedures, double-lumen endotracheal tubes permit ventilation of a single lung and collapse of the lung on the procedural side.

Mapping

Here are maps of three of the cardiothoracic procedures we've discussed:

SURGICAL MAPPING

CABG (coronary artery bypass graft)

Instruments	Important Anatomy Involved	Pathophysiology
Cardiac and Dietrich instrument sets	Heart Coronary blood vessels Sternum	Coronary atherosclerotic heart disease Cigarette smoking Obesity Diet high in saturated fat Hypertension in early age

Microbiology/ Wound Classification	Skin Prep/Incision/ Patient position	Pharmacology
No indigenous microorganism found in the heart Class I (clean)	*Prep:* lower mandible to toes of both legs: bilaterally as far as possible for chest and abdomen and circumferentially for legs *Incision:* from suprasternal notch to xiphoid process *Position:* supine	General anesthesia Heparin Protamine sulfate Cardioplegic solution Epinephrine Lidocaine

SURGICAL MAPPING

Orthotopic heart transplantation

Instruments	Important Anatomy Involved	Pathophysiology
Cardiac and Dietrich instrument sets	Heart Sternum Donor heart	Coronary heart disease Congenital heart failure Valve disease Rejection of previously transplanted heart

Microbiology/ Wound Classification	Skin Prep/Incision/ Patient position	Pharmacology
No indigenous microorganisms in heart Class I (clean)	*Prep:* lower mandible to toes of both legs: bilaterally as far as possible for chest and abdomen and circumferentially for both legs *Incision:* suprasternal notch to xiphoid process *Position:* supine	General anesthesia Heparin Protamine sulfate Cardioplegic solution Epinephrine Lidocaine

Now it's your turn. Use the template available on the Evolve Resources site to try your hand at mapping the remaining procedures:

- Intraaortic balloon pump insertion
- Ventricular assist device (VAD) insertion

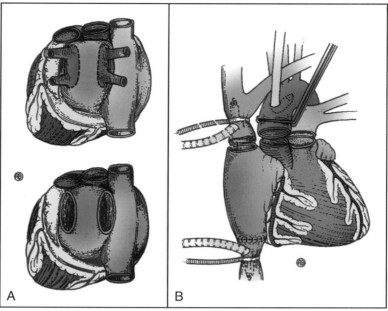

FIG. 7.33 A, Heart transplantation with pulmonary venous anastomoses on right or left side and caval anastomoses at the superior and inferior vena cavae. B, Aorta and pulmonary artery are joined last. (From Waldhausen JA et al: *Surgery of the chest,* ed 6, St Louis, 1996, Mosby.)

SURGICAL MAPPING

Thoracotomy

Instruments	Important Anatomy Involved	Pathophysiology
Thoracotomy instrument set	Ribs Sternum Mediastinum Pleura Lung	Lung tumor

Microbiology/ Wound Classification	Skin Prep/Incision/ Patient position	Pharmacology
No indigenous microorganisms in heart Class I (clean)	*Prep:* from shoulder and axilla to iliac crest and bilaterally as far as possible	General anesthesia

- Valve replacement: aortic, mitral, tricuspid
- Thoracoscopy/VATS (video-assisted thoracoscopy)
- Mediastinoscopy
- Bronchoscopy

NEUROSURGERY

In this section, we'll be reviewing several commonly performed procedures of the nervous system (Fig. 7.34).

Procedures

- Craniotomy
- Ventriculoperitoneal shunt insertion
- Transsphenoidal hypophysectomy
- Laminectomy

- Anterior cervical diskectomy
- Carpal tunnel release
- Ulnar nerve transposition
- Subdural hematoma

Facts to Remember
Craniotomy

- Positioning is crucial in neurosurgery. In each of the following positions, the patient's head is secured with the help of a Mayfield headrest, a three-pin device used to fix the position of the head (Fig. 7.35), or Gardner-Wells tongs:
  - Sitting
  - Beach chair
  - Prone
- Bone wax may be placed on a #4 Penfield dissector for application to control bleeding from the bone.
- A #3 Penfield dissector is used to separate the cranial bone from the dura.
- Raney clips (Fig. 7.36) are applied to control bleeding from the scalp flap.

Laminectomy

See Fig. 7.37 for a typical vertebra.
- Narrowing (stenosis) of the spinal canal can result in chronic pain. In this procedure, the spinous process (**lamina**) is removed, resulting in decompression of the spinal cord and nerve roots.
- Laminectomy is often accompanied by diskectomy.
- The Midas Rex, a high-speed surgical drill, is often used in this procedure.

Anterior Cervical Diskectomy

- Bone is harvested from the iliac crest for grafting.
- The patient is placed in the supine position for this procedure.

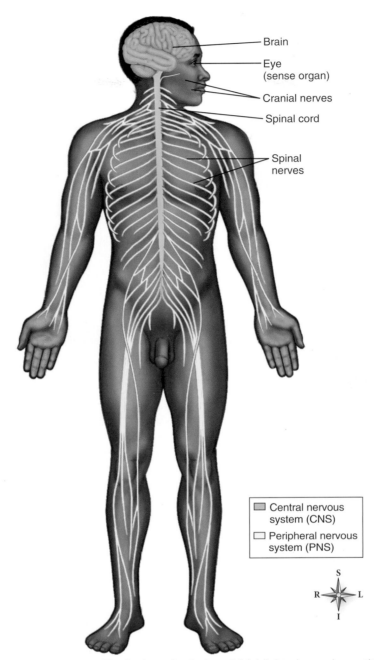

FIG. 7.34 The nervous system. The brain and spinal cord (highlighted green) constitute the central nervous system (CNS), and the nerves (yellow) make up the peripheral nervous system (PNS). (From Patton KT, Thibodeau GA: The human body in health & disease, ed 6, St Louis, 2014, Mosby.)

VP (Ventriculoperitoneal) Shunt

- This procedure (see Fig. 7.38 for a detailed explanation) is performed to alleviate hydrocephalus.
- Two setups—one for craniotomy and the other for laparotomy—are required.
- The wound classification is class I (clean).
- The choroid plexus—located at the fourth, third, and lateral ventricles—produces cerebrospinal fluid (CSF).
- A burr hole is drilled in the occipital or parietal bone, and a ventricular catheter is inserted into the posterior part of the lateral ventricle.

Ulnar Nerve Transposition

- The procedure is indicated for the treatment of cubital tunnel syndrome.
- The nerve is moved to lie under the skin and fat but on top of, within, or under the muscle.
- The ulnar nerve is located behind the medial epicondyle.
- Regional anesthesia (Bier block) is used for this procedure.
- The wound category is class I (clean).

Transsphenoidal Hypophysectomy

Transsphenoidal hypophysectomy (Fig. 7.39) is the surgical removal of the hypophysis (the pituitary gland, also called the

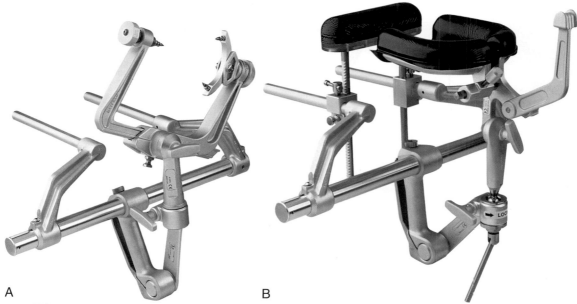

A   B

FIG. 7.35 A, Three-pin fixation skull clamp (Mayfield) for stabilizing head during neurosurgical procedures. **B,** Mayfield horseshoe headrest. (From Rothrock JC: Alexander's care of the patient in surgery, ed 15, St Louis, 2015, Mosby.)

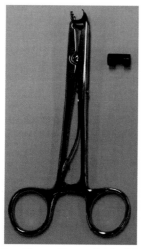

FIG. 7.36 Raney clip. (From Rosenfeld, JV, ed: Practical management of head and neck injury, ed 1, Sydney, 2012, Churchill Livingstone.)

hypophysis) by way of the nose and sphenoidal sinus. It is usually performed in the treatment of tumors, most notably craniopharyngioma, but is also sometimes used in the treatment of Cushing syndrome caused by pituitary adenoma.

- The pituitary gland's location at the base of the cranium makes the nasal approach ideal: The sella (back wall of the sphenoid sinus), consisting of thin bone, lies over the pituitary and can easily be opened to provide access to it. Once the sella has been breached, the surgeon must cut through the dura, the tough inner lining of the skull, to reach the pituitary.

- Once the pituitary gland has been removed, the surgeon patches the hole in the sella with a bone graft taken from the patient's septum. (If the septum is not available—say, if the patient has previously undergone surgery that required it—the surgeon may opt to use synthetic graft material instead.)

A bioadhesive (often referred to as biologic glue) is used to affix the graft material to the hole in the sella. This fosters healing and stops cerebrospinal fluid (CSF) from leaking out of the . This glue allows healing and prevents leakage of the cerebrospinal fluid (CSF) that surrounds the brain out through the damaged sinus and nose.

- Lidocaine with epinephrine is used to after general anesthesia is instilled.

- The wound is categorized as class II (clean contaminated) because of the approach through the nose into the sphenoidal sinus.

Mapping

Here's the mapping for two neurological procedures that you're likely to encounter on your certification exam and in the operating room.

SURGICAL MAPPING

Craniotomy

Instruments	Important Anatomy Involved	Pathophysiology
Craniotomy sets	Cranium	Tumor
	Dura	Epidural or subdural hematoma
		Brain abscess

Microbiology/ Wound Classification	Skin Prep/Incision/ Patient position	Pharmacology
No indigenous microorganisms in brain	*Prep:* area around incision site	General anesthesia
Class I (clean)	*Position:* supine or Fowler	Mannitol
		Topical thrombin

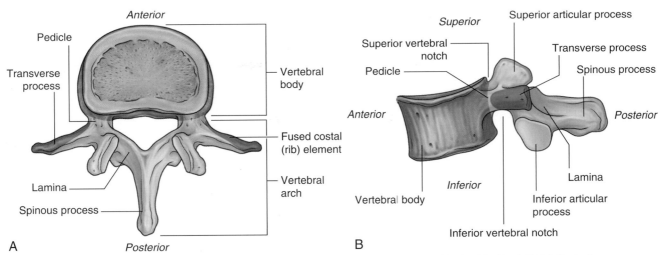

FIG. 7.37 A typical vertebra. **A.** Superior view. **B.** Lateral view. (From Drake RL, Vogl AW, Mitchell AWM: Gray's anatomy for students, ed 3, Philadelphia, 2015, Churchill Livingstone.)

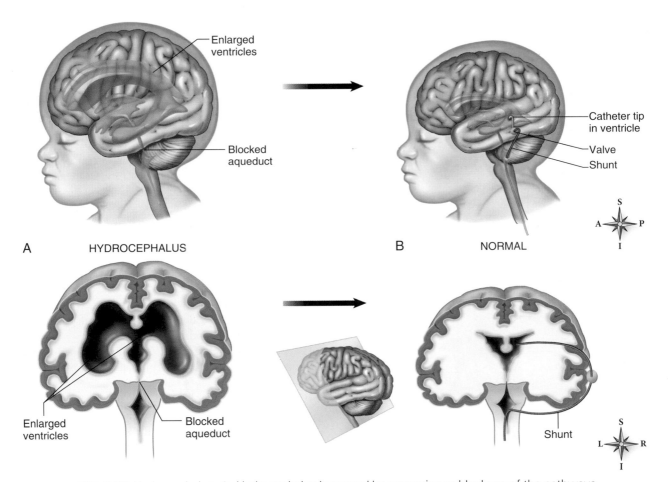

FIG. 7.38 Hydrocephalus. **A,** Hydrocephalus is caused by narrowing or blockage of the pathways for cerebrospinal fluid (CSF), causing the retention of CSF in the ventricles. **B,** This condition can be treated by surgical placement of a shunt or tube to drain the excess fluid. Notice in the cross sections of the brain how the ventricles and surrounding tissue return to their normal shapes and size after shunt placement. (From Patton KT, Thibodeau GA: The human body in health & disease, ed 6, St Louis, 2014, Mosby.)

SURGICAL MAPPING

Laminectomy

Instruments	Important Anatomy Involved	Pathophysiology
Laminectomy set, including these tools: Nerve root (Love) retractor Meyerding retractor Taylor retractor Kerrison rongeur Beckman-Adson retractor	Vertebrae CSF	Disk herniation Lumbar stenosis Lumbar spondylosis

Microbiology/ Wound Classification	Skin Prep/Incision/ Patient position	Pharmacology
No indigenous microorganisms in brain Class I (clean)	*Prep:* depends on which part of spine is affected *Position:* prone	General anesthesia

Using the template available on the Evolve Resources site, try mapping the remaining procedures:
- Ventriculoperitoneal shunt insertion
- Transsphenoidal hypophysectomy
- Anterior cervical diskectomy
- Carpal tunnel release

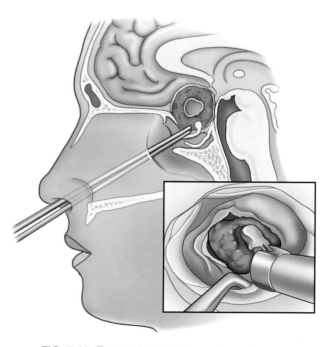

FIG. 7.39 Transsphenoidal hypophysectomy.

- Ulnar nerve transposition
- Subdural hematoma

PLASTIC AND RECONSTRUCTIVE SURGERY

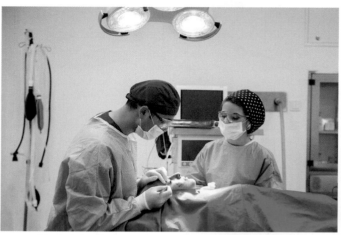

(Copyright © Ozgurdonmaz/iStock/Getty Images.)

The field of plastic surgery comprises two subspecialties:
- Aesthetic surgery, which is also known as *cosmetic surgery*
- Reconstructive surgery, in which provide fundamental needs for social acceptability

The Integumentary System

At the end of every procedure, the main concern for all surgical patients, apart from the success of the treatment, is scarring. For this reason, a thorough understanding of the integumentary system is crucial. Remember that:
- The skin is a sensory organ, registering touch, pressure, pain, and temperature.
- The skin excretes organic water and stores nutrients.
- The epidermis is the outer layer of the skin, and its cells are known as keratinocytes. New epithelial cells begin to push to the surface, where they replace dry and scaly shed cells, by the thousands each days. This process of proliferation and shedding is never-ending.

    Layers of the Epidermis. The Latin word for layer is *stratum* (plural *strata*). The epidermis comprises five *strata* (Fig. 7.40):
- *Corneum* is Latin for "horny": the outer layer of the skin, the **stratum corneum**, consists of dead cells (corneocytes).
- *Lucidum* is Latin for "clear"; the **stratum lucidum**, the next layer down, is a thin layer of dead skin, named for its translucent appearance under a microscope. Commonly found on the palms and soles.
- *Granulosum* is Latin for "small grains"; the **stratum granulosum**, the middle layer of the epidermis, is a thin layer of flattened granular cells.
- *Spinosum* is Latin for "spiny"; the cells of the *stratum spinosum*, the next-to-deepest layer, have a spiky appearance.
- *Basale* is Latin for "base"; the *stratum basale* is the deepest layer of the epidermis.

Skin Grafts

See Fig. 7.41.

Types of Burns

Burns necessitating skin grafts may be inflicted by heat, radiation, friction, chemicals, or electricity.

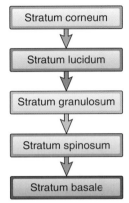

FIG. 7.40 Layers of the epidermis.

Stratum corneum → Stratum lucidum → Stratum granulosum → Stratum spinosum → Stratum basale

First-Degree Burns

- These injuries affecting the epidermis alone.
- They are characterized by mild pain and redness of the skin (erythema).
- Blistering does not occur.

Second-Degree Burns

- Injuries of this type affect the dermis to varying degrees.
- There are two types:
  - Superficial second-degree burns heal within 2 weeks and leave no scar.
  - Deep second-degree burns take longer to heal and leave hypertrophic scarring.

Third-Degree Burns

- In these injuries, the full thickness of the skin and underlying structure are affected.
- If the nerves are damaged, the burned person will feel no pain.
- Burns appear charred or pearly white (eschars).
- A patient with burns of this magnitude is subject to fluid loss and is therefore treated with fluid management, measures to alleviate shock, and sometimes respiratory support.

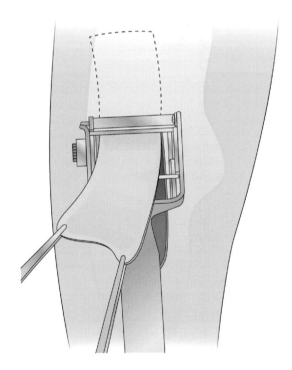

Graft taken from patient's healthy skin

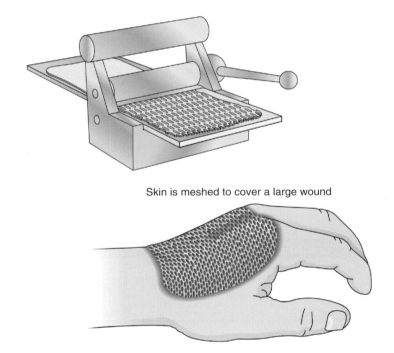

Skin is meshed to cover a large wound

FIG. 7.41 Skin graft technique. A skin graft is a surgical procedure in which a piece of skin is transplanted from one area to another. Often skin will be taken from unaffected areas on the injured person and used to cover a defect, such as a burn. If the area of the skin defect is especially large, the harvested skin may be meshed to stretch it into a larger patch. If the defect involves a great loss of tissue, a full-thickness graft—a flap of skin with underlying muscle and blood vessels—may be required. Taking the graft from the injured person makes rejection of the tissue unlikely. (From Becker JM, Stucchi AF: Essentials of surgery, ed 1, Philadelphia, 2006, Saunders.)

Fourth-Degree Burns

- These injuries are often referred to as *char burns.*
- Only rarely do patients with burns of this severity survive because these injuries are accompanied by catastrophic damage to blood vessels, nerves, muscle, tendon, and sometimes even bone. If a patient with fourth-degree burns does survive, the risk of infection and development of necrosis is high and extensive reconstruction surgery is required.

Procedures

Full-Thickness Skin Graft

- These grafts are performed in cases involving third-degree burns.
- A graft 0.04 inch deep, with a pedicle flap, is harvested.

Split-Thickness Skin Graft

- This type of graft is used in cases of:
  - Superficial second-degree burns (graft thickness 0.02 inch)
  - Deep second-degree burns (graft thickness 0.035 inch)

Additional Facts to Remember

- Before tissue is removed from a donor site, sterile mineral oil or chlorhexidine gluconate is applied with the help of a broad, thin piece of wood (tongue blade). This helps the dermatome glide easily as it is used to harvest skin.
- Certain medications are used to help maintain hemostasis at the donor site. They include:
  - Topical epinephrine
  - Thrombin
  - Phenylephrine
- Once hemostasis is established, a nonadherent gauze is applied:
  - Adaptic + 4×4s
  - Xeroform + 4×4s
  - Opsite
  - Tegaderm
- Tenotomy or iris scissors are used to remove any subcutaneous tissue present in the graft.

Mapping

Here you can see how one kind of skin grafting maps:

SURGICAL MAPPING

Full-thickness skin graft

Instruments	Important Anatomy Involved	Pathophysiology
Plastic instrumentation	Skin	Burns
Dermatome		
Mesher		
Derma-carrier		

Microbiology/ Wound Classification	Skin Prep/Incision/ Patient position	Pharmacology
Class I (clean); burn wounds are sterile in the beginning compared with most wounds	*Donor:* class I (clean) *Recipient:* class II (clean); open wound	General anesthesia

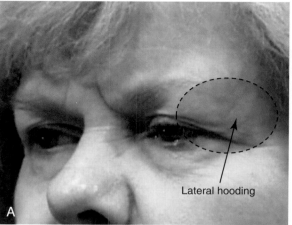

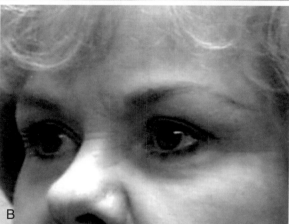

FIG. 7.42 A, A brow lift is required for maximum esthetics in patients with lateral hooding and heavy dynamic glabellar rhytides. B, A 55-year-old woman 6 months following a brow lift and simultaneous upper and lower blepharoplasty. Blepharoplasty or brow lifting alone would probably have been inadequate treatment to fully improve the extreme laxity and lateral hooding. (From Bagheri SC, Bell RB, Khan HA: Current therapy in oral and maxillofacial surgery, ed 1, St Louis, 2012, Saunders.)

Now you try. Using the template available on the Evolve Resources site, map this procedure:
- Partial-thickness skin graft

Head and Face Procedures
Procedures

- Blepharoplasty (eyelid repair or reconstruction; Fig. 7.42)
- Malar implants (cheek implants)
- Mentoplasty (chin augmentation)
- Otoplasty (repair, reshaping, or repositioning of ear)
- Rhinoplasty (repair or reshaping of nose)
- Rhytidectomy (facelift)
- Cleft lip repair
- Cleft palate repair

Facts to Remember

Cheiloplasty/Palatoplasty (Cleft Lip/Palate Repair). Facial development occurs during the first trimester of intrauterine life. One of the most common congenital facial deformities is

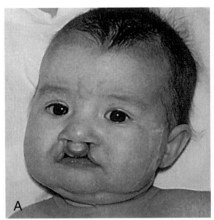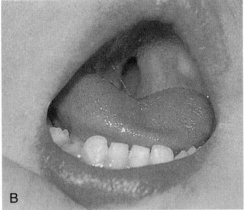

FIG. 7.43 Congenital defects of the mouth. **A,** Bilateral cleft lip in an infant. **B,** Cleft palate. (**A,** From Wilson SF, Giddens JF: Health assessment for nursing practice, ed 2, St Louis, 2001, Mosby. **B,** From Greig JD, Garden OJ: Color atlas of surgical diagnosis, London, 1996, Times Mirror International Publishers.)

cleft lip/cleft palate (Fig. 7.43), in which the parts of the face do not fuse properly during fetal development.

- Surgical intervention for cleft palate is performed when an infant is 11 or 12 months, before facial growth has started; cleft lip repair may be performed at 10 to 12 weeks of age.
- One commonly used type of cheiloplasty is rotation advancement (Millard technique). An incision is made on the edge of the cleft side of the philtrum continued upward, medially, and to the side. A second incision extends to the buccal sulcus (top part of the maxilla). Incision length depends on the size of the gap to be closed. In this second incision, the surgeon frees soft tissue, allowing the lip to be lifted completely from the underlying bone. This dissection should be tested to ensure free advancement toward the middle (inadequate dissection is the root cause of poor results). Nasal deformity can be addressed with a procedure known as McComb nasal tip plasty, in which the depressed nasal dome and rim are elevated. Cartilage from the cleft side is freed from the opposite side, then positioned and reshaped with the use of nylon suture.
- Myringotomy may be performed with this procedure because of the risk of chronic ear infection and partial deafness associated with cleft palate defects.
- The palate is injected with a local anesthetic agent with epinephrine. (Epinephrine, a vasoconstrictor, prolongs the effect of the anesthetic agent and minimizes bleeding.)
- The Dingman mouth gag or cleft palate mouth gag is used during surgery.

Rhytidectomy (Facelift)

- Local anesthetic with epinephrine (as noted just now, a vasoconstrictor) is injected to maintain hemostasis during the procedure.
- Incisions may be made in various areas:
  - Submental (under the chin)
  - Mastoid and neck posteriorly

Mapping

Here you can see how two very different types of facial procedures—cleft repairs and facelift—map.

SURGICAL MAPPING

Cleft lip repair

Instruments	Important Anatomy Involved	Pathophysiology
Plastic instruments sets	Philtrum	Congenital defect
Beaver knife handle and blades	Cupid bow	

Microbiology/ Wound Classification	Skin Prep/Incision/ Patient position	Pharmacology
Indigenous microorganisms in area	*Prep:* area around incision site	General anesthesia
Class II (clean contaminated)	*Position:* supine	

SURGICAL MAPPING

Cleft palate repair

Instruments	Important Anatomy Involved	Pathophysiology
Plastic instruments sets	Philtrum	Congenital defect
Crile-Wood needle holder	Cupid bow	
Freer or Cottle elevator	Hard palate	
	Soft palate	

Microbiology/ Wound Classification	Skin Prep/Incision/ Patient position	Pharmacology
Indigenous microorganisms in area	*Prep:* area around incision site	General anesthesia
Class II (clean contaminated)	*Position:* supine	

Rhytidectomy

Instruments	Important Anatomy Involved	Pathophysiology
Plastic instruments sets	Facial skin	Aging process Excessive exposure to UV light

Microbiology/ Wound Classification	Skin Prep/Incision/ Patient position	Pharmacology
No indigenous microorganisms in area C ass I (clean)	*Prep:* area around incision site *Position:* supine	General anesthesia

Use the template provided on the Evolve Resources site to try mapping the remaining facial procedures:

- Blepharoplasty (eyelid repair or reconstruction)
- Malar implants (cheek implants)

- Mentoplasty (chin augmentation)
- Otoplasty (repair, reshaping, or repositioning of ear)
- Rhinoplasty (repair or reshaping of nose)

Hand Procedures
Procedures
Hand Procedures
- Toe-to-hand transfer (Fig. 7.44)
- Dupuytren contracture repair (subtotal palmar fasciectomy)
- Release of syndactyly (fused digits)

Facts to Remember
- Three nerves supply the hand:
  - Radial nerve
  - Median nerve
  - Ulnar nerve

Mapping
Here we've mapped one reconstructive surgery of the hand. Try it for yourself with the remaining hand procedures:

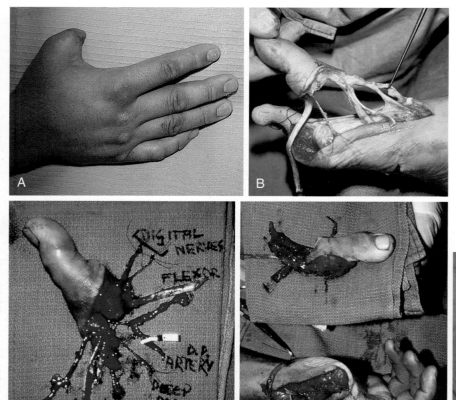
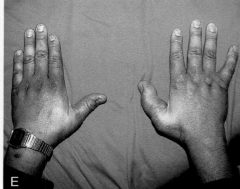

FIG. 7.44 Toe-to-hand transfer. A, Preoperative appearance of hand. B, Harvest of toe. C, Identification of vessels and nerves. D, Transfer of toe to thumb site. E, Postoperative view of toe-to-thumb site transfer. (From Weinzweig N, Weinzweig J: The mutilated hand, St Louis, 2005, Mosby.)

SURGICAL MAPPING
Subtotal palmar fasciectomy

Instruments	Important Anatomy Involved	Pathophysiology
Plastic instruments	Palm	Dupuytren contracture
Minor orthopedic tray	Fourth or fifth digit	

Microbiology/ Wound Classification	Skin Prep/Incision/ Patient position	Pharmacology
No indigenous micro-organism found in the area	From incision site, moving outward to fingertips, up to axillary region	General anesthesia, Bier block, or local sedation
Class I (clean)	Incision on volar or palmar surface of palm or Z-plasty incision	
	Supine	

- Toe-to-hand transfer
- Release of syndactyly (fused digits)

Breast Reconstruction Procedures
Procedures
- Augmentation mammoplasty
- TRAM flap reconstruction (use of abdominal tissue to reconstruct the breast) (Fig. 7.45)
- Mastopexy (repositioning of sagging breasts)

Facts to Remember
- TRAM reconstruction involves the use of a pedicle flap, in which the tissue is harvested along with its blood supply.
- Two setups are required if TRAM flap is scheduled immediately after mastectomy.

- Doppler ultrasound and a sterile probe are used throughout the case to identify the superior and inferior epigastric arteries:
  - The superior epigastric artery is preserved to provide continuous perfusion to the flap.
  - The inferior epigastric artery is double-clamped, cut, and ligated.

Mapping
Here's one of the breast procedures, mapped.

SURGICAL MAPPING
TRAM flap

Instruments	Important Anatomy Involved	Pathophysiology
Basic laparotomy instruments	Breast	Mastectomy
Plastic instruments	Skin and subcutaneous tissue of abdomen	
Dermatome and mesher if skin grafting is indicated for areolar reconstruction	Rectus abdominis muscle	

Microbiology/ Wound Classification	Skin Prep/Incision/ Patient position	Pharmacology
No indigenous microorganisms in area	*Prep:* Neck to midthigh	General anesthesia
Class I (clean)	*Incision:*	
	Elliptical incision from one iliac crest to other; superior incision includes umbilicus; inferior incision is above the pubis symphysis	

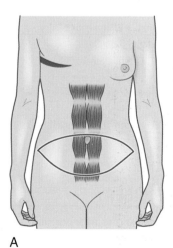 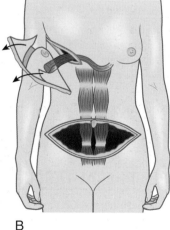 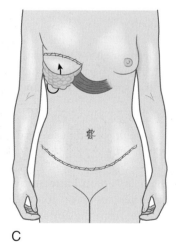 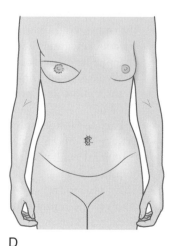

A   B   C   D

FIG. 7.45 Transverse rectus abdominis musculocutaneous (TRAM) flap. **A,** TRAM flap is planned. **B,** The abdominal tissue, while attached to the rectus muscle, nerve, and blood supply, is tunneled through the abdomen to the chest. **C,** The flap is trimmed to shape the breast. The lower abdominal incision is closed. **D,** Nipple and areola are reconstructed after the breast is healed. (From Lewis SL, et al: Medical-surgical nursing: assessment and management of clinical problems, ed 9, St Louis, 2014, Mosby.)

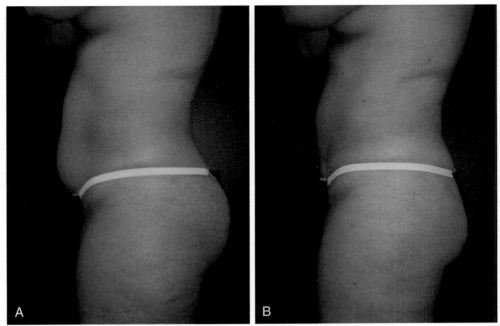

FIG. 7.46 Female 43-year-old patient. **A,** Before and **B,** 6 months after liposuction of the abdomen and buttocks. (From Fortunato N, McCullough SM: Plastic and reconstructive surgery, St Louis, 1998, Mosby.)

Now try it on your own with the remaining breast surgeries:
- Augmentation mammoplasty
- Mastopexy (repositioning of sagging breasts)

Abdominal Procedures
Procedures
- Tumescent liposuction (Fig. 7.46)
- Abdominoplasty ("tummy tuck"; Fig. 7.46)

Facts to Remember
- Tumescent liposuction
  - The tumescent mixture consists of:
    - Lidocaine (anesthetic agent)
    - Epinephrine (vasoconstrictor; maintains hemostasis)
    - Wydase (hyaluronidase; increases permeability and absorption and promotes the spread of local anesthetic)
    - Lactated Ringer solution
  - Extraction of an excessive amount of adipose tissue (>1000 mL) will results in hypovolemia.
- Abdominoplasty
  - This procedure, also known as **panniculectomy**, involves the removal of the **pannus**, an apron-like flap of excess skin and adipose tissue, from the abdominal wall.
  - The patient is maintained in semi-Fowler position to prevent tension on the suture line.

Mapping
Here you see the map for one of these commonly performed plastic surgery procedures.

SURGICAL MAPPING
Tumescent liposuction

Instruments	Important Anatomy Involved	Pathophysiology
Plastic minor Instruments	Any area of the body where subcutaneous fat removal is desired	When diet and exercise fail to cause weight loss

Microbiology/ Wound Classification	Skin Prep/Incision/ Patient position	Pharmacology
No indigenous microorganisms in the area Class I (clean)	Bilaterally, nipple line to midthigh	General anesthesia Tumescent mixture

Now it's your turn. Map the other abdominal plastic surgery procedure:
- Abdominoplasty

PERIPHERAL VASCULAR SURGERY

The peripheral vascular system (Fig. 7.47) is network of vessels that carry oxygenated blood to all areas of the body and then remove the waste products of metabolic processes within the cells.

Overview of the Peripheral Vascular System
Components
- Arteries
- Veins

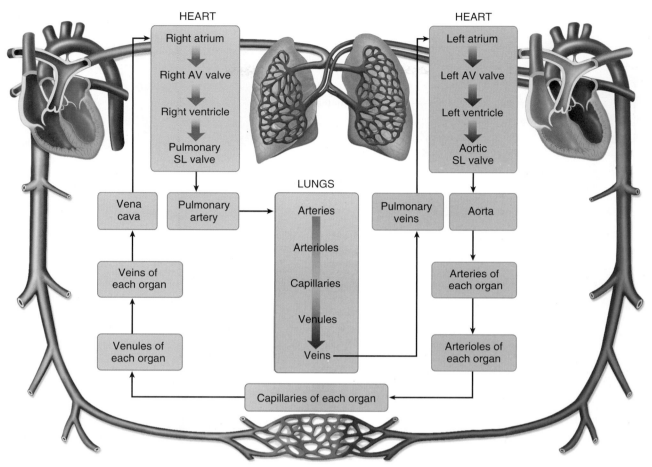

FIG. 7.47 Diagram of blood flow in the cardiovascular system. Blood leaves the heart through arteries, then travels through arterioles, capillaries, venules, and veins before returning to the opposite side of the heart. *AV,* Atrioventricular; *SL,* semilunar. (From Patton KT, Thibodeau GA: The human body in health & disease, ed 6, St Louis, 2014, Mosby.)

- Capillaries
- Venules

Anatomy
- Important blood vessels for review purposes:
  - Abdominal aorta
  - Carotid artery
  - Jugular vessels
  - Internal and external iliac arteries
  - Femoral artery
  - Popliteal artery
  - Venae cavae
- Layers (both arteries and veins)
  - *Tunica adventitia*: outer layer consisting of vaso vasorum, which supplies nutrient to the vessels
  - *Tunica media*: middle layer consisting of smooth muscle that gives it the ability to dilate and contract
  - *Tunica intima*: inner layer of smooth endothelium
- Veins contain valves that prevent backflow of blood
  Table 7.1 and Fig. 7.48 show the main differences between arteries and veins.

TABLE 7.1	COMPARISON OF ARTERIES AND VEINS
Arteries	**Veins**
Thick, elastic walls	Thinner, less elastic walls
No valves	Valves
Blood moves when the heart contracts	Blood moves when skeletal muscle contracts
Pressure is high	Pressure is low
Situated deeper from the surface of the skin	Situated closer to the skin
Injury results in rapid blood loss	Injuries bleed slowly

Physiology
- Blood pressure: Force exerted on the arterial wall by the pumping of heart cycle
- Systole: occurs during the contracture of ventricles
- Diastole: occurs during ventricles are filling and relaxed
- The most common pathophysiologies affecting the peripheral vascular system are arteriosclerosis, atherosclerosis, and thromboembolic disease.

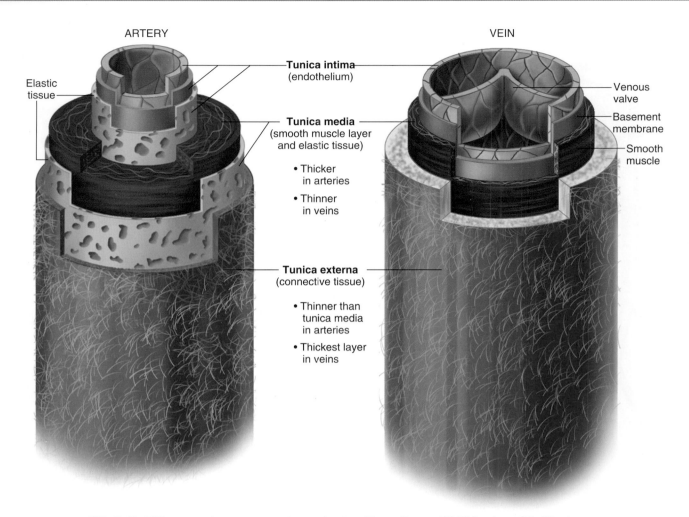

ARTERY

VEIN

Elastic
tissue

Tunica intima
(endothelium)

Venous
valve

Tunica media
(smooth muscle layer
and elastic tissue)

Basement
membrane

Smooth
muscle

• Thicker
in arteries

• Thinner
in veins

Tunica externa
(connective tissue)

• Thinner than
tunica media
in arteries

• Thickest layer
in veins

FIG. 7.48 Differences between arteries and veins. (From Patton KT, Thibodeau GA: The human body in health & disease, ed 6, St Louis, 2014, Mosby.)

Procedures

- Angioplasty
- Embolectomy or thrombectomy
- Abdominal aortic aneurysm (AAA) repair
- Carotid endarterectomy (Fig. 7.49)
- Femoral-popliteal bypass
- Femoral-tibial bypass
- Aorto-femoral bypass
- Arteriovenous fistula and sinus

Additional Facts to Remember
Peripheral Vascular Diagnostic Procedures

- *Arterial plethysmography*
  - This procedure is performed to check blood flow in the arteries of the legs. This is done in people with conditions like hardening of the arteries (atherosclerosis) that causes pain during exercise or poor healing of leg wounds.
  - Three blood pressure cuffs are required: one on each arm and the third on one of the thighs.
  - Each cuff's reading produces a waveform that is then compared with the readings from the other two cuffs

- *Arteriography*
  - This procedure involves the use of contrast medium.
  - Viewing is done with the use of fluoroscopy or CT scan.
  - It is performed before or during surgery or as an interventional procedure.
- *Doppler scanning*
  - This procedure is performed to intensify the sounds of blood flowing in the vessels.
  - The pitch, rhythm and quality of the sound reflect the pressure, volume, and flow rate of the blood.

Peripheral Vascular Surgical Instruments

- *Clamps*
  - Mixter or right-angle clamp
  - Vascular clamps (e.g., DeBakey, Satinsky, Cooley)
- *Scissors*
  - Metzenbaum
  - Potts
  - De Martel
- *Forceps*
  - DeBakey
  - Gerald

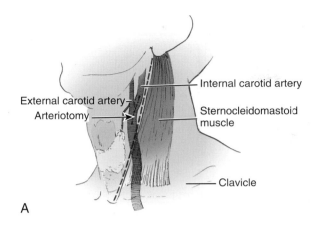

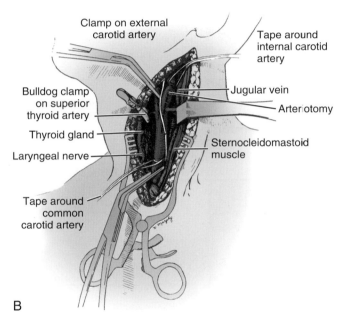

FIG. 7.49 Left carotid endarterectomy. **A,** Incision and anatomy. **B,** Exposure of carotid bifurcation. (From Hershey FB, Calman CH: Atlas of vascular surgery, ed 3, St Louis, 1973, Mosby.)

- *Retractors*
  - Self-retracting
    - Weitlaner
    - Adson-Beckman (articulated tip)
    - Thompson retractor (for abdominal cases, such as AAA [abdominal aortic aneurysm] repair)
  - Handheld
    - Army-Navy
    - Senn
    - Deaver
    - Richardson
- *Suction*
  - Frazier tip
- Blades
  - #11 blade on #7 knife handle

Commonly Used Sutures

Most are double-arm.
- Polypropylene (Prolene)
- Silk
- Gore-Tex

Vascular Graft Materials

- *Autogenous*
  - Saphenous vein
    - Receptive to fine suture technique
    - Easy to tailor
    - Pliable
    - More resistant to infection than synthetic graft material
    - Used in reverse, non-reverse, or *in situ* fashion
    - Easy anastomosis between the proximal end of an artery and the proximal end of the vein because both have larger ends
    - Removal of valves with the use of balloon-tip catheter
- *Synthetic*
  - Knitted polyester
    - Requires pre-clotting because the material is porous and blood tends to seep into it
  - Knitted velour
    - Exoskeleton (EXS) prosthesis
    - Used across the knee
  - Woven polyester
    - Leak-proof
    - Doesn't require pre-clotting by the surgical team
  - Poly-tetra-fluoro-ethylene (PTFE)
    - Used below the knee joint because there is no risk of kinking
    - Rigid rings built in for support

Commonly Used Drugs

- *Heparin*
  - Anticoagulant
  - Protamine sulfate is used for systemic reversal of heparin if the patient is allergic to it or bleeding needs to be restricted.
- *Papaverine*
  - Vasodilator
- *Gelfoam*
  - Absorbable gelatin
- *Thrombin*
  - Of bovine, human plasma, or recombinant DNA origin
  - Mostly added to Gelfoam to initiate the transformation of fibrinogen to fibrin to hasten the clotting process
- *Surgicel*
  - Oxidized cellulose
  - Interacts with blood proteins and platelets
  - Absorbs blood and activates the clotting process
- *Avitene*
  - Collagen of bovine origin
  - Interacts with blood and platelets
  - Absorbs blood and activates the clotting process
- *Contrast media*
  - Omnipaque

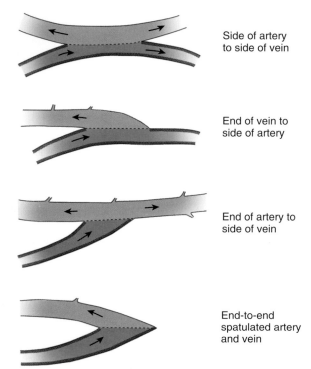

Side of artery
to side of vein

End of vein to
side of artery

End of artery to
side of vein

End-to-end
spatulated artery
and vein

FIG. 7.50 Four types of anastomoses between radial artery and cephalic vein. (From Wilson SE: Vascular access: principles and practice, ed 3, St Louis, 1996, Mosby.)

- Isovue
- Hypaque
- Visipaque

Shunt and Fistula Creation

- If the patient is scheduled for AV shunt surgery, a graft is used.
- If the patient is scheduled for AV fistula surgery, a direct anastomosis between artery and vein is created.
- There are four types of anastomoses (Fig. 7.50):
  - Artery side to vein side
  - Artery end to vein side
  - Artery end to vein end
  - Vein end to artery side
- One shunt procedure performed in the wrist region is the Cimino fistula and shunt (Fig. 8.23).

Carotid Endarterectomy

- Javid or Argyle shunts are placed in the common and internal carotid arteries.
- The plaque is removed with the use of a Freer elevator and Penfield #4 dissector.

Mapping

Here we've mapped two procedures involving parts of the peripheral vascular system:

SURGICAL MAPPING
Arteriovenous fistula or sinus

Instruments	Important Anatomy Involved	Pathophysiology
Vascular instruments DeBakey or Garrett dilator	Radial artery Cephalic vein	Disease necessitating renal dialysis

Microbiology/ Wound Classification	Skin Prep/Incision/ Patient position	Pharmacology
No indigenous microorganisms in the area Class I (clean)	*Prep:* site of incision on the forearm to 3 inches above elbow and to fingertips *Incision:* made over radial artery and cephalic vein *Position:* supine	General anesthesia Heparin Papaverine Gelfoam with thrombin Avitene Surgicel

SURGICAL MAPPING
Carotid endarterectomy

Instruments	Important Anatomy Involved	Pathophysiology
Vascular instruments	Common carotid artery Internal carotid artery	Carotid artery stenosis Resulting TIA (transient ischemic attack)

Microbiology/ Wound Classification	Skin Prep/Incision/ Patient position	Pharmacology
No indigenous microorganisms in area Class I (clean)	*Prep:* starting at site of neck incision on neck to lower border of the ear and to level of axilla *Incision:* anterior line of sternocleidomastoid over carotid bifurcation *Position:* supine, neck hyperextended	General anesthesia Heparin Papaverine Gelfoam with thrombin Avitene Surgicel

And here's one last set of maps for you to complete:
- Angioplasty
- Embolectomy or thrombectomy
- Abdominal aortic aneurysm (AAA) repair
- Femoral-popliteal bypass
- Femoral-tibial bypass
- Aorto-femoral bypass

CONCLUSION

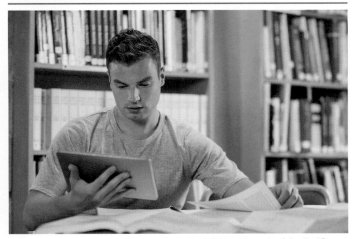

(Copyright © Wavebreakmedia Ltd./Wavebreak Media/Getty Images.)

Congratulations on completing this review of basic surgical procedures! As soon as you feel ready, answer the chapter review questions and check your answers in the Answer Key at the back of the book—but if you feel that you need a bit more work before trying the questions, go back and do some more mapping in any weak areas you've noticed.

REVIEW QUESTIONS

1. Jonathan has been asked to set up an ENT procedure for an injury at the level of the lower segment of the trachea. What other structure at this level could be injured?
   a. Thoracic aorta
   b. Esophagus
   c. Thymus
   d. Mediastinum

2. A surgeon is teaching a resident how to perform an appendectomy. The resident asks the name of the surgical incision. What is it?
   a. McBurney
   b. Paramedian
   c. Oblique
   d. Transverse

3. When setting up for a gastrectomy procedure, the surgical technologist should add vascular instruments for the specific purpose of ligating the:
   a. Treitz arterial stump
   b. Branches of the peritoneal artery
   c. Popliteal artery
   d. Splenic vessels

4. Surgical excision of the pylorus with end-to-end anastomosis of the stomach and duodenum is called:
   a. Billroth II
   b. Billroth 1
   c. Gastrectomy
   d. Duodenostomy

5. A 50-year-old patient in an ambulatory surgical center OR bed has been positioned in the jackknife position. Which procedure requires this positioning?
   a. Sigmoidectomy
   b. Hemorrhoidectomy
   c. Spinal fusion
   d. Removal of rectal foreign body

6. Which statement about the liver, spleen, and pancreas is true?
   a. All three are solid organs and very vascular.
   b. All three organs are involved in immune function.
   c. All three organs are involved in metabolism.
   d. All of these statements are false.

7. The primary function of the gallbladder is to:
   a. Convert bile salts into bile enzymes
   b. Manufacture bile
   c. Contract to secrete bile into the hepatic duct
   d. Store and concentrate bile

8. The Whipple procedure is:
   1. Removal of the head of the pancreas
   2. Removal of the entire duodenum
   3. Removal of part of the jejunum
   4. Removal of the distal third of the stomach
   5. Removal of the lower half of the common bile duct
   6. Partial gastrectomy
      a. 1, 2, 3, 4, 6
      b. 1, 2, 3, 4, 5, 6
      c. 1, 3, 5, 6
      d. 1, 2, 4, 5

9. What are the boundaries of the Hesselbach triangle?
   a. Rectus abdominis muscle, Cooper ligament, transverse colon
   b. Inguinal ligament, rectus abdominis muscle, deep epigastric vessels
   c. Inguinal ligament, epigastric artery Cooper ligament
   d. Camper fascia, epigastric vessels, external oblique muscle

10. The ducts located on each side of the lower end of the vagina that secrete mucus are known as:
    a. Bartholin glands
    b. Perineal glands
    c. Labial glands
    d. Skene glands

11. A woman is scheduled for endometrial ablation. What is the ideal surgical position for this procedure?
    a. Prone
    b. Sims
    c. Lithotomy
    d. Supine

12. Herniation of the rectum to the vaginal vault is called:
    a. Rectocele
    b. Dermoid cyst
    c. Cystocele
    d. Hydrocele

13. In this procedure, a suture ligature is placed around the cervix to prevent spontaneous abortion.
    a. Cerclage
    b. Eclampsia
    c. Myomectomy
    d. Dilation and curettage

14. The surgeon wants to dilate a patient's urethra for transurethral resection of the prostate. What dilator is preferred for this procedure?
    a. Hagar dilators
    b. Van Buren sounds
    c. Uterine sounds
    d. Bake dilator

15. Vesicourethral suspension (Marshall-Marchetti-Krantz procedure) is a suspension of the bladder neck and urethra to the cartilage of the pubic symphysis to treat urinary stress incontinence in the female. Which incision is the ideal approach to permit entry of the Retzius space?
    a. Lower midline or Pfannenstiel
    b. Midline epigastric
    c. Upper midline incision
    d. Transurethral

16. Epispadias is a rare condition in which the urethral meatus is located:
    a. At the base of the penis
    b. On the lateral side of the penis
    c. On the inferior side of the penis
    d. On the top side of the penis

17. In _____, an opening is made surgically in the tympanic membrane to release fluid from the middle ear.
    a. Mastoidectomy
    b. Tympanoplasty
    c. Myringotomy
    d. Stapedectomy

18. Which of these instruments is not used in tonsil and adenoid surgery?
    a. Crowe-Davis gag
    b. Tonsil snare
    c. Scissors
    d. Babcock forceps

19. Cerumen is more commonly known as:
    a. Earwax
    b. Keratin
    c. Cholesteatoma
    d. Polyp

20. During total shoulder arthroplasty, the humeral head and _____ are replaced with artificial components to restore function and relieve pain. In hemiarthroplasty, only the humeral component is replaced.
    a. Glenoid capsule
    b. Scapula
    c. Clavicle
    d. Biceps

21. The epiphyseal plate is a hyaline cartilage plate in the metaphysis at each end of a long bone. This plate is also known as the:
    a. Growth plate
    b. Diaphyseal plate
    c. Periosteum
    d. Shaft

22. One example of a sesamoid bone is the:
    a. Tibia
    b. Patella
    c. Hyoid
    d. Olecranon

23. The Bankart and Putti-Platt procedures are performed to:
    a. Treat rheumatic arthritis
    b. Surgically repair fractures of the proximal humerus
    c. Correct recurrent anterior dislocation of the shoulder
    d. Restore stability to the shoulder joint and alleviate pain

24. Which type of fracture is common in children?
    a. Open
    b. Spiral
    c. Transverse
    d. Greenstick

25. Which muscle is **not** part of the rotator cuff?
    a. Supraspinatus
    b. Teres minor
    c. Infraspinatus
    d. Deltoid

26. In the Cloward method, a special dowel cutter is used to take a plug of bone from the _____ to serve as a bone graft.
    a. Iliac crest
    b. Rib
    c. Clavicle
    d. Ulna

27. Which procedure is performed to evacuate intracranial hematomas, tumors, or vascular lesions that are not accessible through a burr hole?
    a. Craniectomy
    b. Craniosynostosis
    c. Cranioplasty
    d. Craniotomy

28. The glossopharyngeal, trigeminal, and trochlear nerves are all:
    a. Spinal nerves
    b. Facial nerves
    c. Cranial nerves
    d. Collateral nerves

29. A Le Fort II fracture:
    a. Starts at the nasal bones, crosses the frontal process of the maxilla and lacrimal bones, and extends laterally along the maxillary sinus wall
    b. Starts at the nasal bones, crosses the frontal process of the maxilla and lacrimal bones, and extends through the orbital floor, infraorbital rim, and lateral maxillary sinus wall
    c. Starts at the frontal process of the maxilla and lacrimal bones and extends through the orbital floor, infraorbital rim, and lateral maxillary sinus wall
    d. Starts at the nasal bones, crosses the frontal process of the maxilla and lacrimal bones, and extends through the lateral maxillary sinus wall

30. The TRAM flap is described as:
    a. A free flap
    b. A pedicle-based flap
    c. Mastopexy
    d. A rotated, tunneled flap

31. Facelift is also known as:
    a. Rhytidectomy
    b. Cheiloplasty
    c. Blepharoplasty
    d. Septoplasty

32. Augmentation of the chin is known as:
    a. Mentoplasty
    b. Le Fort I repair
    c. ORIF
    d. Cheiloplasty

33. What type of graft is skin harvested from same individual's body?
    a. Homograft
    b. Heterograft
    c. Xenograft
    d. Autograft

34. Dupuytren disease is a condition that causes contraction of the:
    a. Palmar fascia
    b. Aponeurosis
    c. Dorsum of the hand
    d. Plantar fascia

35. How many extraocular muscles are found in each eye?
    a. Four recti and two oblique muscles
    b. Two superior muscles and one lateral muscle
    c. Two inferior and two medial muscles
    d. Two recti and four oblique muscles
36. Removal of the entire orbital contents, including the periosteum, for certain malignancies of the globe or orbit is known as:
    a. Evisceration
    b. Exclusion
    c. Exenteration
    d. Enucleation
37. The procedure performed to remove the eyeball when the eye muscles and optic nerve been severed is called:
    a. Exenteration
    b. Evisceration
    c. Keratoplasty
    d. Enucleation
38. A 70-year-old man complains that he is losing his vision. Examination reveals that the crystalline lenses of both eyes are opaque. What surgery does the ophthalmologist schedule?
    a. Enucleation
    b. LASIK
    c. Capsulorrhexis
    d. Cataract removal
39. Strabismus surgery is performed to:
    a. Correct deviation of the eye
    b. Repair the optic nerve
    c. Correct paralysis of the levator palpebrae muscle
    d. Correct deficient nerve stimulation
40. Mydriatric drugs such as _____ are used to dilate the pupil.
    a. Phenylephrine
    b. Naloxone
    c. Hyaluronidase
    d. Lidocaine
41. Thyroidectomy (surgical removal of all or part of the thyroid gland) is used in the treatment of malignancy or hyperthyroidism. Which instruments should be available in the event of bilateral cord paralysis?
    a. General surgery minor set
    b. Vascular set
    c. Plastic set
    d. Tracheotomy set
42. What are the names of the three small articulating bones in the ear?
    a. Anvil, head, and hammer
    b. Ossicles, incus, and crura
    c. Stapes, capitulum, and stirrup
    d. Malleus, incus, and stapes
43. The largest salivary gland is the:
    a. Zygomatic
    b. Parotid
    c. Submandibular
    d. Sublingual
44. Which of the three layers of the eye is found near where the iris and sclera join? (The incision is made through this layer for vitrectomy.)
    a. Iris layer
    b. Pars plana layer
    c. Tapetum lucidum
    d. Cornea
45. All intraocular gases used to flatten a detached retina and keep it attached during the healing process are mixed with sterile air **except**:
    a. Sulfur hexafluoride (SF6)
    b. Perfluoroethane (C2F6)
    c. Nitrous oxide
    d. Perfluoropropane (C3F8)
46. Piggyback transplantation of the heart is also known as:
    a. Heterotopic transplantation
    b. Orthotopic transplantation
    c. Hemi-transplantation
    d. Double transplantation
47. All of these nerves supply the hand **except** the:
    a. Ulnar nerve
    b. Brachial nerve
    c. Median nerve
    d. Radial nerve
48. Which of these statements about veins is true?
    a. The walls are thick and elastic.
    b. Blood moves when the heart contracts.
    c. Pressure is high.
    d. Blood moves when skeletal muscle contracts.
49. The tunica media consists of:
    a. Endothelial muscle
    b. Smooth muscle
    c. Skeletal muscle
    d. Columnar muscle
50. What kind of graft material is used below the knee joint because it carries no risk of kinking. (It has rigid rings built for support.)
    a. Polytetrafluoroethylene (PTFE)
    b. Knitted polyester
    c. Knitted velour
    d. Woven polyester

Answers for this exam and an electronic version of the exam can be found in the Answer Key at the back of the book.

1. During a craniotomy, what medication might be needed to reduce intracranial pressure?
   a. Epinephrine
   b. Lidocaine
   c. Dantrolene
   d. Mannitol

2. The _____ self-retaining retractor provides the best exposure in thoracotomy.
   a. Balfour
   b. Gelpi
   c. Weitlaner
   d. Finochietto

3. Maria the CST, setting up for TURP, selects _____ as the medium for distention because it is _____.
   a. NACL; electrolytic
   b. H_2O; hypotonic
   c. Lactated Ringer solution; neutral
   d. Glycine; non-electrolytic

4. Which cranial nerve is it important to preserve during rhytidectomy?
   a. X
   b. V
   c. VII
   d. I

5. Donna the CST is preparing the room for a patient with a hip fracture. She knows that the patient will be placed in the _____ position and that _____ will be needed during the procedure.
   a. Lateral with beanbag; x-ray
   b. Lateral with fracture table; C-arm
   c. Supine with beanbag; traction
   d. Supine with fracture table; C-arm

6. Pablo, the CST in Room 4, knows that Creutzfeld-Jakob disease can be caused by exposure to _____ during neurological procedures _____ and that surgical instruments that are suspected of having come in contact should be _____.
   a. Staphylococci; sterilized
   b. DIC; destroyed
   c. Streptococci; sterilized
   d. Prions; destroyed

7. With which of these pathogens is the diabetic patient most susceptible?
   a. *Bacillus subtilis*
   b. *Treponema pallidum*
   c. *Clostridium perfringens*
   d. *Escherichia coli*

8. Jack, the CST on call, knows that standard precautions should be implemented:
   a. For HIV patients
   b. In emergency procedures only
   c. Whenever blood and body fluids may be encountered
   d. In accordance with hospital policy

9. Tracy, the CST in the scrub role, is stuck with a contaminated needle during a surgical procedure. Which of these microorganisms can be transmitted through needlesticks?
   a. *Mycobacterium tuberculosis*
   b. *Staphylococcus albus*
   c. *Pseudomonas aeruginosa*
   d. *Hepatitis B virus*

10. Dawn, a CST, is preparing for an arteriography. Which of these contrast media is most likely to be used in this procedure?
    a. Methylene blue
    b. Hypaque
    c. Gentian violet
    d. Indigo carmine

11. A patient undergoing a surgical intervention suffers a malignant hypothermia (MH) crisis. The anesthesiologist will most likely administer:
    a. Dantrolene and succinylcholine
    b. Propofol, furosemide
    c. Furosemide, dantrolene
    d. Naloxone, furosemide

12. The patient in room 5 is undergoing pilonidal cystectomy. In what position will the patient be placed?
    a. Lateral
    b. Supine
    c. Prone
    d. Lithotomy

13. During an appendectomy, the surgeon exposes the appendix and is ready to grasp it. Which instrument should the CST in the scrub role anticipate that the surgeon will request?
    a. Kocher clamp
    b. Babcock forceps
    c. Allis clamp
    d. Heaney clamp

14. The surgical team is preparing to transfer a patient with a fractured femur from the traction bed to the OR table. Who is responsible for maintaining the fracture's position during the transfer?
    a. Anesthesiologist
    b. Registered nurse
    c. Circulating CST
    d. Surgeon

15. The CST in the scrub role is setting up the sterile field for an open hernia operation when she notices that a Gelpi retractor has perforated the back table cover. The best plan of action is:
    a. Discarding the retractor and covering the area with a towel
    b. Discarding the retractor and covering the area with sterile drapes
    c. Discarding the retractor, saving all the sterile instruments she can, and setting up a new back table
    d. Breaking down the entire field and establishing a new one

16. What is the best site at which to apply the dispersive electrode during laparotomy?
    a. Buttocks
    b. Calf
    c. Thigh
    d. Clipped to the drapes

17. During a surgical procedure, a team member touches the nonsterile IV pole. The CST in the scrub role should:
    a. Notify the surgeon
    b. Notify the supervisor
    c. Remove the team member's contaminated glove and reglove him
    d. Tell the team member to have the circulator remove the glove

18. The case in room 4 is a LAVH. In what position does the CST anticipate that he will need to place the patient?
    a. Prone
    b. Lateral
    c. Fowler
    d. Lithotomy

19. While draping a patient for repair of a right inguinal hernia, Raquel, the CST in the scrub role, notices an exposed area of unprepped skin. The best choice of action for the surgical team is to:
    a. Break down the setup, re-prep, and re-drape
    b. Slide the already placed drape up to cover the area
    c. Slide the already placed drape down to cover the area
    d. Cover the area with a new drape

20. The degree of humidity in the operating room is directly related to:
    a. The team's comfort
    b. Well-being of pediatric patients
    c. Use of anesthesia gases
    d. Presence of static electricity

21. All of the following surgical procedures require three surgical counts except one that requires four. Which surgery requires four counts?
    a. Total hip arthroplasty
    b. CABG
    c. Liver transplant
    d. Cesarean section

22. Heather, the CST in the scrub role, anticipates that the surgeon will need thermal hemostasis. What is her best choice for this method?
    a. Thrombin
    b. Heparin
    c. Silver nitrate
    d. Monopolar cautery

23. In the middle of a surgical procedure, the surgeon requests a larger self-retaining retractor for exposure of the abdomen, and the CST in the scrub role requests that the Bookwalter retractor be opened. Before using this retractor, the CST must:
    a. Arrange instruments
    b. Ask surgeon which pieces will be used
    c. Verify that the retractor will fit the wound
    d. Count each piece individually

24. In an ACL _____ reconstruction, the surgeon plans to harvest the patient's _____.
    a. Xenograft; biceps tendon
    b. Allograft; Achilles tendon
    c. Synthetic graft; broad ligament
    d. Autograft; patellar tendon

25. During a procedure, Tim, the CST in the scrub role, is conducting the closing count with the circulator, and they find a discrepancy. They each recount again and find that they are still missing an item. How should they proceed?
    a. Calling the x-ray department
    b. Notifying the supervisor
    c. Breaking scrub and looking in the garbage
    d. Notifying the surgeon and stopping the closure

26. Tina, the CST in room 3, has finished a procedure and is preparing the instrumentation for decontamination. She should:
    a. Unlock all instruments in a basin filled with NaCl solution
    b. Lock all instruments and place them in a basin filled with water
    c. Place the instruments in basin, then unlock them and spray then with enzymatic cleaner
    d. Not clean any unused instruments

27. The primary use of retention sutures in wound closure is:
    a. As an aid in wound healing
    b. Primary closure
    c. Prevention of dehiscence
    d. To provide exposure

28. The autoclave tape on a wrapped sterilized item indicates whether an item:
    a. Has been exposed to the process of sterilization
    b. Is nonsterile
    c. Is contaminated
    d. Is sterile

29. Which spore is used to monitor and guarantee that the sterilization process has taken place in the steam autoclave?
    a. *Geobacillus stearothermophilus*
    b. *Bacillus staphylococcus*
    c. EtO
    d. Hydrogen peroxide

30. When preparing for procedures in patients with severe burn injuries, the CST should remember that:
    a. Pain medication may be needed
    b. Extra irrigation may be required
    c. Extra wound dressing may be required
    d. Intact skin is the body's first defense against infection

31. Which lab value would be of concern to a surgical team performing a TAH?
    a. Hemoglobin 8–10
    b. RBC 5,000,000
    c. WBC 7000
    d. Hematocrit 34%–44%

32. The main reason for the use of the Sellick maneuver by the CST in the circulating role is:
    a. To help anesthesia intubate
    b. To help position the endotracheal tube
    c. To help ensure dental integrity
    d. To help prevent aspiration

33. When picking up a patient for transport to the OR, the CST must complete all of the following tasks **except**?
    a. Confirming that this is the correct patient
    b. Ensuring that the stretcher is locked
    c. Ensuring that all jewelry has been removed
    d. Having the patient sign the consent form

34. Which action would invalidate the informed consent for surgery?
    a. The nurse explains the procedure to the patient.
    b. The CST serves as a witness to the consent.
    c. The surgeon obtains consent.
    d. An illiterate patient signs with a mark.

35. A patient who has just undergone surgery explains to the nurse that the surgeon has told her that her wound will heal by granulation. In which phase of wound healing does this occur?
    a. Class I
    b. Class III
    c. Class II
    d. Class IV

36. Which of these conditions does **not** contribute to poor wound healing?
    a. Diabetes
    b. Early ambulation
    c. Malnutrition
    d. Obesity

37. *Res ipsa loquitur* is a Latin term concerning:
    a. Patient rights
    b. The AST motto
    c. Doing no harm
    d. Negligence

38. The surgeon finishes a hernia operation and breaks scrub. The CST is applying a sterile dressing when the surgeon realizes that he has forgotten to give the postoperative pain injection and asks the CST to complete this task. The CST indicates that she may not because:
    a. It would be negligence
    b. Anesthesia will have to do it
    c. No consent has been issued to the CST
    d. It would be malpractice

39. All of the following are sentinel events that would result in the creation of an incident report **except**:
    a. Patient burn
    b. Drug error
    c. Calling in sick
    d. Improper handling of a specimen

40. The schedule indicates that the patient in room 6 is to undergo laparoscopic cholecystectomy with cholangiogram. The CST should anticipate the need for:
    a. Blood replacement
    b. Two setups
    c. Lead apron and thyroid shield
    d. Chest drainage system

41. CST Dave is preparing to scrub for an abdominal aortic aneurysm repair in room 7. He should open his gown and gloves:
    a. The back table near the corner
    b. On the Bovie machine
    c. On the linen hamper
    d. On a separate prep table

42. A CST preparing for a procedure involving the use of a laser should be aware of all of these safety precautions except:
    a. Use of a halon fire extinguisher against laser fire
    b. Use of a smoke evacuator to remove the plume
    c. Use of laser safety glasses only for individuals who do not wear glasses
    d. Posting of warning signs on doors of ORs in which lasers will be used

43. Jackie, a CST working 7 AM to 3 PM, is scrubbed in on a laminectomy at 3 PM. Her relief is going to be about 10 minutes late. Jackie decides to leave anyway to pick her daughter up at school. She could be liable for:
    a. Negligence
    b. Malpractice
    c. Abandonment
    d. Accountability

44. Julie, working in central supply, is preparing a scope for high-level disinfection. She knows that _____ is a high-level disinfectant and also a sterilant.
    A. Alcohol
    B. Glutaraldehyde (Cidex)
    C. Carbolic acid (phenol)
    D. Povidone-iodine (Betadine)

45. CST Lisa is an expert on aseptic technique. She knows that all of these procedures are sterile except:
    a. Mediastinoscopy
    b. Pelvic laparoscopy
    c. Colposcopy
    d. TMJ arthroscopy

46. During a procedure, the CST in the scrub role is asked by two sterile residents scrubbed in on the procedure whether they can safely change position. The CST tells them to pass each other:
    a. Front to back
    b. Side to side
    c. Front to front or back to back
    d. Back to front

47. In positioning the sterile back table in accordance with aseptic technique, the CST knows that the table should be placed _____ from the unsterile wall.
    a. 2 feet
    b. 5 inches
    c. ½ foot
    d. 12 to 18 inches

48. A CST and RN in room 4 setting up for a 10 AM colon resection have counted and are prepared to receive the patient when they are informed that the surgeon will be 20 minutes late. The pair decides to go take a coffee break and locks the OR to preserve the setup. When they return from break, the setup is no longer sterile. Why?
    a. Someone entered the room
    b. Their break was too long for the setup to remain sterile
    c. Unguarded sterile fields are considered contaminated
    d. They should have turned the air off

49. Dr. Ortiz has a rotator cuff repair scheduled in room 4. When she arrives in the room, she sees the sterile CST sitting on a stool. She informs the CST that they must break and rescrub because:
    a. The CST is too close to the floor
    b. The CST has altered his level of sterility
    c. The CST can never sit without compromising sterility
    d. She needs the stool for positioning

50. While completing an ACL reconstruction in room 5, the surgeon drops the locking graft screw on the floor. When the surgeon tells the nurse to flash the screw for use, the CST informs the surgeon that they may not do this, because:
    a. There is no consent
    b. Flash is for emergencies only
    c. The screw is contaminated
    d. Implants can never be safely flash-sterilized

51. All of the following actions could invalidate a surgical consent **except**:
    a. Medicating the patient before obtaining the signature
    b. Coercing the patient
    c. Informing the patient of the risks and benefits
    d. Poor mental health of patient

52. The CST should help position the patient undergoing a D&C by:
    a. Raising one leg at a time to place them in the stirrups
    b. Ensuring that the buttocks are positioned below the midline position of the bed
    c. Raising the legs simultaneously to place them in the stirrups
    d. Crossing the arms over the chest

53. The primary concern of the surgical team using DuraPrep or a one-step prep application for a surgical procedure is:
    a. Pressing hard with the applicator
    b. Ensuring that the entire area is covered
    c. Allowing pooling of solution
    d. Ensuring that the prep solution is given adequate drying time

54. A surgeon performing an odontectomy gives the CST permission to pass the specimen off the field. The CST knows that specimens containing stones & teeth should be sent:
    a. In a container with moist Telfa
    b. In a container with formalin
    c. In a container with NaCl solution
    d. In a dry container

55. In preparing for a pediatric surgical intervention, the CST should:
    a. Request a longer booking time for procedure
    b. Anticipate the need for increased irrigation fluids
    c. Request a cryotherapy unit
    d. Anticipate the use of warming devices (e.g., Bair Hugger)

56. All of these findings are indications of impending MH crisis **except**?
    a. Increase in temperature
    b. Unexplained tachycardia
    c. Muscle rigidity
    d. Decreased CO_2 level

57. To eliminate anticipated dead space, what might the surgeon request?
    a. Montgomery straps
    b. Pressure dressing
    c. Extra suture material
    d. Postoperative injection

58. A patient who has just undergone cholecystectomy contracts an infection and is brought back to the OR for irrigation and debridement. What wound classification is assigned to the second procedure?
    a. Class I
    b. Class II
    c. Class III
    d. Class IV

59. Dr. Diaz, performing a cholecystectomy, tells the CST that he will need a drain for the common bile duct. The CST should anticipate the need for a:
    a. Penrose drain
    b. T-tube
    c. Tenckhoff catheter
    d. Levin tube

60. In anticipation of gastric spillage during gastrectomy, the surgeon might ask the anesthesiologist to insert a:
    a. Foley catheter
    b. A-line
    c. Red rubber Robinson catheter
    d. Salem sump tube

61. At the end of a CYSTO procedure, the surgeon asks Luna the CST to send the stones to pathology for analysis. Luna should send the specimen:
    a. In a dry specimen container
    b. For frozen analysis
    c. For culture
    d. On a moist RayTec sponge

62. A patient undergoing cystectomy generally has an ileal conduit procedure as well. The stoma is created from the:
    a. Sigmoid colon
    b. Kidney
    c. Ascending colon
    d. Ileum

63. During a pyelolithotomy procedure, a medical student asks the surgical technologist why a silk suture may not be used to repair the ureter. The CST replies that:
    a. It is not listed on the preference card
    b. The surgeon likes to use nonabsorbable monofilament sutures
    c. Silk is only used in vascular procedures
    d. Silk is contraindicated in the genitourinary system

64. A pediatric patient has been found to have strabismus. Which equipment will the CST likely have on his Mayo setup?
    a. Rat tooth forceps, Potts-Smith scissors
    b. Bayonet forceps, speculum
    c. 0.12-mm forceps, Army/Navy retractor
    d. Calipers, muscle hook

65. Students are watching as the CST in room 4 organizes the sterile field for the next procedure. The CST is labeling mineral oil and placing cotton balls and a dermatome in a corner of his back table. He is mostly likely preparing for:
    a. Breast implant insertion
    b. Full-thickness skin grafting
    c. Rhytidectomy
    d. Split-thickness skin grafting

66. While preparing the fixation instrumentation for a hip fracture, Miguel the CST overhears the surgeon stating that she will use a dynamic hip screw for fixation. The steps that Miguel should anticipate for screw insertion are:
    a. Tap, drill, measure, screw
    b. Drill, countersink, tap, screw
    c. Drill, measure, tap, screw
    d. Measure, drill, tap, screw

67. In which position will a patient most likely be placed for total hip arthroplasty?
    a. Prone
    b. Supine
    c. Fowler
    d. Lateral

68. All of the following bones are involved in triple arthrodesis **except** the:
    a. Talus
    b. Ilium
    c. Navicular bone
    d. Calcaneus

69. During carotid endarterectomy, the CST should ensure that one of these items is on the sterile field for the procedure. Identify the item.
    a. Doppler ultrasound
    b. T-tube
    c. Penrose drain
    d. Javid shunt

70. During vascular procedures, the CST in the scrub role should expect the surgeon to use _____ to prevent vasospasm.
    a. Heparin
    b. Thrombin
    c. Cross-clamping
    d. Papaverine

71. The surgeon has requested an active drain for a patient undergoing mastectomy. The CST should ask the circulator for a?
    a. Chest drainage system
    b. Penrose drain
    c. Salem sump tube
    d. Hemovac drain

72. During exploratory laparotomy, the CST overhears the surgeon say that the patient will need a colon resection and anastomosis. The CST should prepare the sterile field for:
    a. Vascular instrumentation
    b. Preparation of a frozen section specimen
    c. Bowel isolation technique
    d. Multiple abdominal incisions

73. During colon resection, the surgeon removes the tumor from the splenic flexure. The CST in the scrub role should expect the surgeon to create an anastomosis between the _____ and the _____.
    a. Duodenum; ascending colon
    b. Cecum; descending colon
    c. Ileum; sigmoid colon
    d. Transverse colon; descending colon

74. To ensure patient safety during laparoscopic cholecystectomy, the CST should:
    a. White-balance the camera
    b. Ensure that the insufflator is set at 20 mm
    c. Place a grounding pad on the patient's back after placing her in the lithotomy position
    d. Instructing the circulator to place light source on standby when the scope is outside the abdomen

75. Dr. Smith's preference card calls for a blunt trocar and dissection down to the peritoneum for his laparoscopic approach. Which piece of equipment will not be used in this procedure?
    a. Veress needle
    b. 10-mm trocar
    c. Insufflation tubing
    d. 5-mm trocar

76. Dr. Rex has scheduled a patient in room 6 for repair of a retinal detachment and has requested the use of a laser. The CST knows that laser most commonly associated with this type of repair is the:
    a. CO_2
    b. Harmonic scalpel
    c. Argon
    d. Krypton

77. Which scissors would most likely be used for dissection during strabismus surgery?
    a. Metzenbaum
    b. Jorgenson
    c. Tenotomy
    d. Westcott

78. During anterior pelvic exenteration the CST must anticipate an additional procedure. What is it?
    a. Nephrectomy
    b. Ileal conduit
    c. Rectocele
    d. Myomectomy

79. Gibson and flank incisions are possible approaches for procedures involving the:
    a. Uterus
    b. Colon
    c. Kidney
    d. Pilonidal cyst

80. A CST participating in a TURP procedure knows that at the end of the case the surgeon will insert a _____ catheter to promote hemostasis.
    a. Fogarty
    b. Red rubber Robinson
    c. Jackson Pratt
    d. Three-way Foley

81. A CST in the scrub role expects the surgeon performing suprapubic prostatectomy to make:
    a. An umbilical incision
    b. The Pfannenstiel incision
    c. A perineal incision
    d. An inguinal incision

82. A patient has had a finding of a torn labrum. The surgical intervention most likely to be performed is?
    a. Knee arthroscopy
    b. TAH
    c. Bankart procedure
    d. Colporraphy

83. Which tendon is most likely to be harvested from a patient undergoing ACL repair?
    a. Quadriceps
    b. Biceps
    c. Patellar
    d. Achilles

84. The pathologic condition most commonly associated with total knee arthroplasty is:
    a. Rheumatoid arthritis
    b. Osteomyelitis
    c. Osteoarthritis
    d. Osteoporosis

85. While scrubbing for cerebral aneurysm clipping, CST Diego recalls that the anatomic structure that is probably involved is the:
    a. Subclavian artery
    b. Fourth ventricle
    c. Circle of Willis
    d. Choroid plexus

86. During mastoidectomy, the surgeon uses a nerve stimulator to identify the:
    a. Facial nerve (cranial nerve VII)
    b. Vagus nerve (cranial nerve X)
    c. Trigeminal nerve (cranial nerve V)
    d. Vestibulocochlear nerve (cranial nerve VIII)

87. During cerebral aneurysm clipping, the surgeon applies a clip, but it does not cover the entire base of the defect. The surgeon removes the clip and hands it back to the CST, who then:
    a. Reloads the clip
    b. Discards the clip
    c. Prepares a suture instead
    d. Prepares a Gore-Tex graft

88. The patient in room 6 is scheduled for ventriculoperitoneal shunt placement. The distal end of the shunt may be placed in the peritoneum or the right atrium. The proximal end of the shunt should be placed in the:
    a. Dura mater
    b. Cerebellum
    c. Ventricle
    d. Pia mater

89. The patient in room 8 is scheduled for anterior cervical diskectomy and fusion. To fuse the cervical disk space, the surgeon will most likely harvest bone from the:
    a. Clavicle
    b. Bone bank
    c. Iliac crest
    d. Cervical lamina

90. The surgeon has asked for the reamer to smooth out the glenoid. What procedure is most likely being performed?
    a. Rotator cuff repair
    b. Hip fracture
    c. Total shoulder arthroplasty
    d. Laminectomy

91. When draping the patient for a D&C procedure, the first drape to be placed is the:
    a. Legging
    b. Abdominal
    c. Under buttock
    d. Sticky towels

92. The circulator is preparing to prep the patient for a STSG. The surgeon indicates that he will harvest the STSG from the left thigh and implant the graft in to the right thigh. The best choice for prepping is:
    a. Prepping the right side first
    b. Prepping the left side, then draping
    c. Prepping the left side first and separately, then prepping the right side with a second prep set
    d. Prepping both sites at the same time, splitting the prep tray in two

93. Marco, a CST in room 4, is in the middle of a colon resection and asks the circulator for more NaCl. The circulator begins to pour the NaCl into the basin at the corner of the sterile back table when the cap falls from her hand onto the corner of the back table. What is the best plan of action for the CST in the scrub role?
    a. Telling the surgeon to give antibiotics
    b. Isolating and covering the contaminated area with sterile towels
    c. Breaking down the entire back table
    d. Calling the supervisor to file an incident report

94. During laparoscopic oophorectomy, the CST should expect the surgeon to request that the patient be placed in the:
    a. Trendelenburg position
    b. Fowler position
    c. Sims position
    d. Reverse Trendelenburg position

95. George, the CST in the circulating role, is helping position the patient for pilonidal cystectomy. All of the following positioning equipment is necessary **except**?
    a. Chest rolls
    b. Antiembolic devices
    c. Arm boards
    d. Beanbag

96. While the staff is conducting the initial count, before the patient is brought into the room, a fly lands on the back table. The best choice of action is to:
    a. Cover the area with sterile towels and eliminate the fly
    b. Spray alcohol at the fly
    c. Turn off the room lights and open the OR door
    d. Break down the table and retrieve a new setup

97. A patient who recently underwent abdominal surgery presents in the emergency department with separation of the wound edges and protrusion of the viscera. The diagnosis is:
    a. Herniation
    b. Dehiscence
    c. Dead space
    d. Evisceration

98. The elimination of dead space is a priority for the surgical team. All of the following are good ways to eliminate dead space **except**?
    a. Allowing separation of the wound layers
    b. Inserting a drain
    c. Applying a pressure dressing
    d. Using proper suturing techniques

99. The term granulation is usually associated with _____ wound closure.
    a. Delayed
    b. Primary
    c. First intention
    d. Secondary intention

100. All of the sterile technique principles listed below are correct **except**?
    a. If in doubt, throw it out
    b. The back of a sterile gown is considered unsterile.

c. Sterile drapes, once placed, may be adjusted as needed.
d. Movement around the sterile field should be kept to a minimum.

101. All of the following should be counted on the sterile field **except**?
    a. Tonsil sponges
    b. Kitners
    c. Cottonoids
    d. Dressing sponges

102. The tissue that surrounds and protects the kidney is the:
    a. Gleason capsule
    b. Glomerulus
    c. Gerota fascia
    d. Hilum

103. A patient presents in the preoperative area for total knee arthroplasty. The following lab results are attached to the patient's chart. Which finding is cause for concern?
    a. Hemoglobin 14 g/dL
    b. White blood cell count of 11,000/mm^3
    c. Partial thromboplastin time of 14 seconds
    d. Hematocrit of 42%

104. Incorrect labeling, loss, or other mishandling of a surgical specimen by a CST or the circulator could result in a charge of:
    a. Malpractice
    b. Negligence
    c. Larceny
    d. Abandonment

105. Only one of the agents listed below can function as a high-level disinfectant for 20 minutes and as a sterilant for 10 hours. Which is it?
    a. Peracetic acid
    b. Isopropyl alcohol
    c. Glutaraldehyde
    d. Hydrogen peroxide

106. Of the situations listed below, which constitutes a break in sterile technique?
    a. The white cuff of a sterile team member's gown is covered by her gloves.
    b. A sterile team member sits for a procedure that will be performed with the staff sitting.
    c. A nonsterile team member maintains a 6-inch distance from the sterile field.
    d. A nonsterile team member applies a dispersive electrode.

107. Sharps safety is always a priority for the surgical team. Which of these actions indicates a need for education on sharps safety?
    a. Never recapping hypodermic needles
    b. Using a needle counter for a procedure that involves one suture
    c. Establishing a neutral zone within the sterile field
    d. Banging on the side of the sharps container when it is full to make extra space

108. The CST should know that all of the following are breaks in sterile technique **except**?
    a. Gowning off a separate table
    b. Covering a sterile back table for use in another OR
    c. Considering a surgical gown sterile from waist to the midchest line in front
    d. Pulling a suction tip that falls below the table's edge back onto the field

109. The hemostatic agents listed below are all applicable to the sterile field, but only one is contraindicated for parenteral use. Which is it?
    a. Collagen
    b. Silver nitrate
    c. Thrombin
    d. Gelfoam

110. Staff members who will be involved in hemolytic transfusions must know that the universal donor blood type is _____ and that the universal recipient blood type is _____.
    a. A; O
    b. B; AB
    c. A; B
    d. O; AB

111. Malignant hyperthermia can be triggered by succinylcholine. Signs include increased metabolic state and increased temperature. The anesthesiologist administers two medications to counter MH. What are they?
    a. Dantrolene and furosemide
    b. Xylocaine and morphine
    c. Furosemide and Levophed
    d. Demerol and Lasix

112. At the end of a knee arthroscopy procedure, the surgeon requests a steroid for injection to control swelling. The CST in the scrub role should expect to draw up:
    a. Demerol
    b. Xylocaine
    c. Dexamethasone
    d. Marcaine

113. During CABG the surgeon requests a medication that will act as a vasodilator. The CST should expect to draw up:
    a. Epinephrine
    b. Thrombin
    c. Heparin
    d. Papaverine

114. The main reason for the application of the Sellick maneuver is to:
    a. Help anesthesia see
    b. Prevent laryngospasym
    c. Facilitate intubation
    d. Prevent aspiration

115. The suture of choice for anastomosis in the femoral popliteal bypass procedure is:
    a. Chromic
    b. Double-armed polypropylene
    c. Vicryl
    d. Silk

116. All of the following are acceptable practices of aseptic technique and preservation of the sterile field **except**:
    a. Maintaining the sterile field until the patient is transported to the PACU
    b. Monitoring the sterile field for breaks in technique
    c. Ensuring that unsterile personnel maintain a distance of 12 to 18 inches from the sterile field
    d. Going on coffee break only if no one is in the OR and the doors are locked

117. During the perioperative process, the circulator is responsible for all of the following tasks **except**:
    a. Prepping the patient
    b. Verifying the correct patient
    c. Caring for specimens
    d. Organizing the sterile field

118. Most surgical departments are built in a racetrack design. The department is also delineated by restricted, semi-restricted, and unrestricted areas. An individual who is wearing scrubs, hat, and booties would be allowed to enter the:
    a. Sterile storage
    b. Operating rooms
    c. Restricted area
    d. Semi-restricted area

119. To prevent microemboli with the use of PMMA during total hip arthroplasty, what might the surgeon use before the PMMA is applied?
    a. Cement restrictor
    b. Antibiotics
    c. Caulking gun
    d. Pulse lavage

120. During thoracotomy, the surgeon requests a clamp to grasp the lung tissue. The CST in the scrub role prepares to hand the surgeon:
    a. Kelly forceps
    b. Duval forceps
    c. Lahey forceps
    d. Mixter forceps

121. On examining a patient, the surgeon notes an acquired inguinal hernia that presents within the Hesselbach triangle. The diagnosis is;
    a. Femoral hernia
    b. Umbilical hernia
    c. Indirect hernia
    d. Direct hernia

122. A Penrose drain is used during the inguinal hernia repair to:
    a. Provide drainage
    b. Aid in the repair
    c. Retract the spermatic cord
    d. Retract the inferior epigastric artery

123. The surgeon has requested that 500 mg of Ancef be added to 1000 mL of NaCl for irrigation. The circulator shows you the vial of Ancef, which reads, "250 mg/mL." How much should you draw up?
    a. 1 mL
    b. 1000 mL
    c. 2 mL
    d. 3 mL

124. The Billroth procedure is most commonly associated with malignancy. The CST should be prepared for the possibility of seeding and the anatomy associated with the:
    a. Kidneys
    b. Bladder
    c. Larynx
    d. Stomach

125. Vagotomy is performed in people with gastric ulcers and gastric secretion issues. The procedure involves ligation of cranial nerve:
    a. V
    b. I
    c. IX
    d. X

126. Laparoscopic appendectomy requires the establishment of pneumoperitoneum to create a safe working environment. The appendix is transected and the stump closed through the use of:
    a. The purse-string suture
    b. Ligaclips
    c. Linear cutters
    d. LDS stapling

127. A patient who has just undergone colon resection presents with a fever and increased WBC count. The CST on the first case did not implement adequate bowel isolation technique. The microbe most likely associated with this infection is:
    a. *Clostridium perfringens*
    b. Creutzfeld-Jakob disease prion
    c. Methicillin-resistant *Staphylococcus aureus*
    d. *Escherichia coli*

128. All of these statements regarding the heart are true **except**:
    a. The right atrium receives deoxygenated blood from the vena cava.
    b. The left atrium receives oxygenated blood from the pulmonary vein.
    c. The left ventricle pumps deoxygenated blood into systemic circulation.
    d. The right ventricle pumps deoxygenated blood to the pulmonary artery.

129. The surgeon in room 10 has requested the use of a device that cuts and cauterizes tissue by means of ultrasonic energy. The CST asks the circulator to set up the:
    a. Bipolar cautery
    b. Monopolar cautery
    c. Harmonic scalpel
    d. Argon beam

130. The emergency procedure underway in room 6 requires a mini drill. None is available. The minimum time exposure for a drill is:
    a. 3 minutes
    b. 5 minutes
    c. 30 minutes
    d. 10 minutes

131. The responsibility of obtaining informed consent for emergency appendectomy lies with the:
    a. RN
    b. Anesthesiologist
    c. CST
    d. Surgeon

132. Semi-Fowler position is appropriate for patients in all of these surgical interventions except:
    a. Bankart
    b. Craniotomy
    c. Mastectomy
    d. Colporrhaphy

133. To ensure patency of the femoral artery during a bypass procedure, what should the CST in the scrub role have on the sterile field?
    a. Pulse oximeter
    b. Capnography machine
    c. Sphygmomanometer
    d. Doppler

134. The surgeon's preference card calls for 60 mg of heparin, and the vial the circulator presents to you reads, "30 mg/mL." How much do you draw up?
    a. 4 mL
    b. 1 mL
    c. 2 mL
    d. 0.5 mL

135. Class IV wounds have the highest infection rate. All of the following situations are categorized as class IV except:
    a. Gross spillage stomach during gastrostomy
    b. Incision and drainage of abscess
    c. 4-hour-old gunshot wound
    d. Delayed primary closure

136. The drain that should be associated with choledochotomy the:
    a. Pezzer
    b. Salem sump
    c. T-tube
    d. Penrose

137. The surgeon performing a myomectomy explains to a student that the tumors are benign and that they are found in the muscle layer, called the:
    a. Endometrium
    b. Myocardium
    c. Epicardium
    d. Myometrium

138. For practical purposes during craniotomy, the CST in the scrub role should perform all of the following tasks **except**?
    a. Keeping track of the amount of irrigation used
    b. Preparing Raney clips for use on the scalp
    c. Using hot NaCl solution for irrigation
    d. Prepare for seeding isolation technique when malignancy is discovered

139. A patient with a tumor of the pituitary gland will probably be scheduled for:
    a. Nephrectomy
    b. Thyroidectomy
    c. Transsphenoidal hypophysectomy
    d. Total abdominal hysterectomy

140. For which of these surgical interventions should the CST have a tracheostomy tray available in the room during the procedure?
    a. Laryngoscopy
    b. Thoracotomy
    c. Pneumonectomy
    d. Thyroidectomy

141. The landmark that is essential for the surgeon performing intramedullary femur rodding is the?
    a. Acetabulum
    b. Diaphysis of the femur
    c. Femoral head
    d. Greater trochanter

142. A patient in the emergency department is found to have a Colle fracture. The CST on call knows that the surgeon can fix this type of fracture by means of closed reduction or open reduction and internal fixation (ORIF). This fracture involves the:
    a. Tibia
    b. Humerus
    c. Radius
    d. Ulna

143. The patient in room 6 has stress incontinence. The surgeon informs the surgical team that this will be an open repair. The procedure on the schedule should state:
    a. Colporraphy
    b. Stamey procedure
    c. MMK
    d. Cysto TURBT

144. For the AAA repair procedure in room 6, the CST should ensure that all of the following equipment is available **except**?
    a. Doppler
    b. Auto transfusion machine
    c. Aneurysm clips
    d. Dacron graft material

145. Don is preparing for a procedure in a patient who has abnormal enlargement of the veins of the spermatic cord. The procedure he is preparing for is:
    A. Vasovasotomy
    B. Inguinal hernia repair
    C. Hydrocelectomy
    D. Varicocelectomy

146. An arteriovenous fistula is an abnormal joining of a vein and an artery. The indication for this procedure is dialysis. The best choice for artery and vein anastomosis is the:
    a. Radial artery and cephalic vein
    b. Brachial artery and saphenous vein
    c. Femoral artery and vena cava
    d. Carotid artery and subclavian vein

147. During AAA repair, the surgeon asks for a vascular clamp to occlude the aorta. The CST prepares to pass a:
    a. Bulldog clamp
    b. Allen clamp
    c. Heaney clamp
    d. Satinsky clamp

148. For the CST working with a surgeon who is performing rhytidectomy, a practical consideration is ensuring preservation of the:
    a. Cephalic vein
    b. Cranial nerve X
    c. Cranial nerve V
    d. Cranial nerve VIII

149. In mentoplasty, the surgeon can choose from various types of implant material, including silicone, Teflon, and autograft. The draping for this procedure includes:
    a. Extremity draping
    b. A pediatric lap sheet
    c. Stockinette
    d. Head and neck draping

150. The cochlear implant procedure involves the implantation of a device in the temporal bone. The procedure is performed to treat sensorineural deafness. Which cranial nerve does it involve?
    a. VII
    b. Median
    c. II
    d. VIII

151. FESS surgical intervention is performed to treat conditions that inhibit normal breathing. The sinuses that are located between the eyes and are related to this procedure are the:
    a. Maxillary
    b. Sphenoid
    c. Frontal
    d. Ethmoid

152. When preparing for a keratoplasty in room 6, the CST should ensure that the donor grafts are in the room and that the _____ is on the sterile field.
    a. Nerve stimulator
    b. Doppler
    c. Phacoemulsification handpiece
    d. Trephine

153. When performing an intracapsular cataract extraction procedure, the CST should anticipate the need for materials not used for the extracapsular cataract extraction procedure, including:
    a. A phacoemulsification unit
    b. An I&A unit
    c. Healon
    d. 8-0 suture material

154. Dacrocystorhinostomy involves the anatomy of the:
    a. Bladder
    b. Uterus
    c. Lacrimal sac
    d. Ovaries

155. Hysteroscopy involves the insertion of a hysteroscope into the cervix. Before insertion, which dilator does the surgeon use to create space for the scope?
    a. Bakes
    b. Van Buren
    c. Debakey
    d. Heager

156. The CST in the cysto room is working with the surgeon on a cysto TURP. The surgeon needs to evacuate the prostatic chips that are obstructing his view. The CST anticipates the need for:
    a. Irrigation
    b. Van Buren sounds
    c. Ellik evacuator
    d. Resectoscope

157. In an abdominal perineal resection, the CST should anticipate the need for patient positioning in the lithotomy position and two separate sterile fields. What else will be needed?
    a. Vascular tunneler
    b. EEA
    c. Randall forceps
    d. Bennett retractor

158. For the approach on a lumbar laminectomy, the surgeon has asked for a self-retaining retractor with ratcheted arms. The CST should pass the surgeon a:
    a. Weitlaner retractor
    b. Gelpi retractor
    c. Finochietto retractor
    d. Beckman retractor

159. The pathology associated with radical neck dissection and mandibulectomy is malignancy of the mouth and jaw. The CST working on this procedure should anticipate the possible need for two sterile setups and graft harvesting. The most likely site of graft procurement for this procedure is the:
    a. Iliac crest
    b. Femur
    c. Humerus
    d. Fibula

160. When working on an emergency tracheostomy, the CST in the scrub role should prepare the Mayo stand for immediate use of items. The CST should also:
    a. Wait to open the tracheostomy tube to ensure the correct size
    b. Have a Poole suction tube available on the field
    c. Ensure patency of the tube balloon
    d. Have sterile Doppler ultrasound available

161. In preparation for the LEEP procedure, the CST in the scrub role organizes the kit. The CST encounters Monsel solution, which is used for hemostasis, and another solution that will be used for the Schiller test. What is it?
    a. Xylocaine
    b. Betadine
    c. Hypaque
    d. Lugol

162. When readying a patient for D&C, the CST in the circulating role should begin the prep at the:
    a. Umbilicus
    b. Thighs
    c. Pubic area
    d. Abdomen

163. While performing laparoscopic cholecystectomy, the surgeon requests an endo bag. The main purpose of this device is:
    a. Facilitating closure
    b. Containing the specimen and avoiding spillage
    c. Protecting the sterile field from the x-ray tech
    d. Facilitating cholangiography

164. The CST who is on call is assigned an emergency splenectomy. The CST should expect to see heavy blood loss and the use of the autotransfusion device and vascular clamps. After surgery, the patient will have?
    a. Improved circulation
    b. Increased metabolism
    c. A weakened immune system
    d. Resistance to antibiotics

165. All of the following procedures require the patient to be placed in the lithotomy position **except**:
    a. Excision of a Bartholin cyst
    b. Vulvectomy
    c. Abdominal perineal resection
    d. Vasovasotomy

166. Gram staining is an essential tool for the lab to identify bacteria. Cultures of specimens obtained from a patient are stained, and the color indicates whether a bacterium is gram positive or gram negative. A gram-positive bacterium is _____, and a gram-negative one is _____.
    a. Blue; pink
    b. Yellow; blue
    c. Black; blue
    d. Pink; blue

167. Frozen section specimens are sent off the sterile field immediately and taken to the lab. Specimens should never be sent:
    a. On Telfa
    b. In a jar alone
    c. Labeled
    d. On a RayTec sponge

168. All of the following clamps are intestinal clamps and can be used to facilitate intestinal anastomosis **except** the:
    a. Allen clamp
    b. Dennis clamp
    c. Lahey clamp
    d. Doyen clamp

169. For the CST scrubbing on an oral and maxillofacial procedure, patency of the airway is essential, and the CST should remember to:
    a. Have Bakes dilators available
    b. Have a vascular tray on standby
    c. Include a throat pack in the count
    d. Have sterile Doppler ultrasound available to assess patency

170. In STSG, the equipment that will be needed to expand the surface area of skin harvested from the thigh is:
    a. The dermatome
    b. Mineral oil and a tongue depressor
    c. Bovie electrocautery
    d. The mesh graft device

171. The circulator is preparing and positioning a patient scheduled for an LAVH in room 6. The best site for placement of the dispersive electrode is the:
    a. Back
    b. Thigh
    c. Buttock
    d. Forearm

172. An Esmarch tourniquet is used to exsanguinate a limb and help reduce blood loss. This equipment is used all of these surgical procedures **except**:
    a. Total knee arthroplasty
    b. ORIF of ankle
    c. Carpal tunnel release
    d. ORIF of hip

173. Inferior vena cava filter insertion can be accomplished by way of two approaches, the femoral approach and the jugular approach. The main goal of this procedure is to:
    a. Restore circulation
    b. Prevent hypoxia
    c. Shunt blood flow
    d. Prevent pulmonary embolism

174. When working on peripheral vascular procedures, the CST is aware of the possibility of embolus formation. To deal with this possibility, José ensures that _____ catheters are in the room.
    a. Foley
    b. Pezzar
    c. Fogarty
    d. Groshong

175. In most vascular procedures, heparin is administered to the patient to prevent the formation of blood clots. Once the procedure is complete, the surgeon might request that _____ be administered to the patient to reverse the effects of the heparin.
    a. Naloxone (Narcan)
    b. Protamine sulfate
    c. Vitamin k
    d. Papaverine

ANSWER KEY FOR CHAPTER REVIEW QUESTIONS

CHAPTER 1

1. B. Hysterectomy is surgical removal of the uterus.
2. B. The suffix *-ia* means "pain."
3. B. The prefix *supra-* means "above."
4. D. The acronym ORIF stands for "open reduction and internal fixation."
5. D. The suffix *-itis* means "inflammation."
6. B. Gastrectomy is removal of all or part of the stomach.
7. C. The suffix *-megaly* means "enlargement," so *cardiomegaly* means "enlargement of the heart."
8. A. The prefix *dys-* means "painful" or "abnormal."
9. D. *TAH/BSO* stands for "total abdominal hysterectomy and bilateral salpingo-oophorectomy," referring to removal of the entire uterus and both ovaries and fallopian tubes.
10. C. The suffix *-necrosis* refers to death of a tissue.
11. C. *Chondr/o* is the root word referring to cartilage.
12. C. The prefix *ad-* means "near" or "toward"; therefore the surgeon is asking the CST to move the patient's arm closer to the body.
13. A. The root word *kerat/o* refers to the cornea of the eye, and the suffix *-plasty* refers to surgical repair of a body part. Keratoplasty is the surgery in which a diseased or damaged cornea is replaced with a healthy donor cornea.
14. D. The root word *myring/o* refers to the tympanic membrane, and the suffix *-otomy* means "the act of making an incision." Therefore myringotomy is a procedure in which a cut is made into the eardrum.
15. A. The suffix *-oma* means "tumor."
16. A. An opening made by a surgeon from the outside of the body into the ileum, part of the small intestine, is known as an ileostomy.
17. D. The suffix *-scopy* denotes the use of a scope to view something, and the root word *arthr/o* refers to the joints, so arthroscopy is the use of a scope to view the inside of a joint.
18. B. The surgery used to repair cryptorchidism is known as orchiopexy, which means "the fixation of a testicle."
19. B. The suffix *-rrhaphy* means "suturing." Herniorrhaphy is the term for hernia repair.
20. A. *Otoplasty* (root word *oto*, meaning "ear," and suffix *-plasty*, meaning "repair") is the term for surgical repair of the ear.
21. C. *Hypertrophy* (root word *trophy*, meaning "growth," and prefix *hyper-*, meaning "excessive) is the term for excessive, unusual, or pathological growth of an organ or structure.
22. C. The instrument used to cut bone is an osteotome (root word *osteo*; suffix *-tome*, meaning "cutting instrument.")
23. A. Eschar is dead matter that is cast off from the skin's surface after a burn.
24. C. A thrombus is a mass of undissolved matter that may be found in a blood or lymphatic vessel. Emboli may be solid, liquid, or gaseous in form.
25. B. *Effusion* is the term used to describe the escape of fluid into a part or area of the body.

CHAPTER 2

1. B. Endocardium lines the inner wall of the heart chambers. It consists of cells that are embryologically and biologically similar to the endothelial cells that line blood vessels. The endocardium also provides protection to the valves and heart chambers.
2. B. The sinoatrial node, the heart's natural pacemaker, is found on top of the right atrium.
3. D. Cardiac contraction is the result of electrical stimulation of the heart muscle.
4. C. Electrical stimulation or impulse spreads through the atria in a wavelike motion. When the contraction reaches the bottom of the right atrium, it stimulates an area of special tissue called the atrioventricular node. This takes the impulse from the atria and passes it on to the ventricles, traveling through the bundle of His, bundle branches, and Purkinje fibers in the muscle of the ventricles. When the stimulation reaches the ventricles, a ventricular contraction occurs.
5. B. The tricuspid valve is located between the right atrium and right ventricle.
6. A. The aortic valve is located between the left ventricle and the aorta.
7. D. The mitral valve is located between the left atrium and left ventricle.
8. C. In regurgitation, the valve doesn't close completely, allowing blood to flow backward through it. This results in leakage of blood back into the atria from the ventricles (in the case of the mitral and tricuspid valves) or leakage of blood back into the ventricles (in the case of the aortic and pulmonary valves).
9. A. In atresia, the valve opening hasn't developed at all, preventing blood from passing from an atrium, to a ventricle or from a ventricle to the pulmonary artery or aorta. Blood must find an alternate route, usually through another existing congenital (present at birth) defect, such as an atrial septal defect or a ventricular septal defect.
10. B. The submucosa is the thick connective tissue layer containing blood vessels, small glands, and the submucosal nerve plexus.
11. D. The greater omentum is the mesentery that connects the greater curvature of the stomach to the transverse colon and posterior body wall. The parietal peritoneum is the serous membrane that covers the interior surface of the body wall.
12. C. The stomach is not a retroperitoneal organ. The retroperitoneal organs comprise the duodenum, pancreas, ascending colon, descending colon, rectum, kidneys, adrenal glands, and urinary bladder.
13. D. The frenulum is a thin fold of tissue that is part of the tongue. It anchors the tongue anteriorly to the floor of the mouth.

14. B. Adults normally have 32 permanent teeth; children have 20 deciduous teeth.

15. A. The center of the tooth, called the pulp, is filled with blood vessels, nerves, and connective tissue.

16. B. Dentin is the living cellular and calcified tissue that surrounds the pulp cavity.

17. C. Amylase is secreted by the pancreas and salivary glands.

18. A. *Palatine* is not the name of one of the three pairs of extrinsic salivary glands.

19. D. Bile is produced by hepatocytes in the liver and then secreted into the bile canaliculi.

20. A. The main part of the stomach is known as the body of the stomach.

21. D. The primary responsibilities of the large intestine are the compaction, storage, and elimination of feces.

22. B. Salivary amylase begins the digestion of carbohydrate molecules.

23. C. The stomach is home to the smallest number of bacteria.

24. D. The gastrointestinal wall surrounding the lumen of the gastrointestinal tract is made up of four layers of specialized tissue. From outside to inside, these layers are the serosa, the muscular layer, the submucosa, and the mucosa.

25. C. The appendix is located at the cecum, which is part of the ascending colon.

26. B. *Escherichia coli* produces vitamin K.

27. B. The gallbladder is located in the angle between the right costal margin and the linea semilunaris, usually on the transpyloric plane, but it may be found as low as the iliac crest.

28. D. The pancreas, an exocrine and endocrine gland, has a head, neck, body, and tail. The portal vein is formed posterior to the neck of the pancreas by the union of the superior mesenteric and splenic veins.

29. C. Pyloric stenosis is a congenital disorder in which the pylorus is thickened, resulting in obstruction of the gastric outlet to the duodenum. This problem is more common in boys. The symptoms, including projectile vomiting, appear several weeks after birth.

30. B. The splenorenal ligament is the peritoneal structure that connects the spleen to the posterior abdominal wall over the left kidney. It also contains the tail of the pancreas. The gastrocolic ligament connects the greater curvature of the stomach with the transverse colon. The gastrosplenic ligament connects the greater curvature of the stomach with the hilum of the spleen. The phrenicocolic ligament connects the splenic flexure of the colon to the diaphragm. Finally, the transverse mesocolon connects the transverse colon to the posterior abdominal wall.

31. C. The esophagus lies posterior to the trachea.

32. A. The opening in the diaphragm that allows the esophagus to pass through and connect to the stomach is known as the esophageal hiatus.

33. C. Kidney cells produce the hormones renin and erythropoietin, but their primary function is excretion of body waste.

34. B. The skin is the largest organ in the human body.

35. C. Melanin is responsible for both skin and hair color.

36. C. A third-degree burn affects the epidermis and dermis. This patient is a candidate for full-thickness skin grafting.

37. C. The pulmonary artery carries deoxygenated blood. (The pulmonary vein carries oxygenated blood.)

38. D. The tunica adventitia is the outer layer of a blood vessel. The tunica media is the middle layer. The tunica intima is the innermost layer.

39. B. In the systole phase, the ventricles contract, pumping blood to the arteries. In the diastole phase, the ventricles are relaxed and the heart fills with blood.

40. C. The innermost layer of the uterus is the endometrium. The middle layer of the uterus is the myometrium. The outermost layer of uterus is the perimetrium. There is no such thing as the epimetrium.

41. D. In women, the erectile tissue that corresponds to the corpus spongiosum in men is the clitoris.

42. D. The primary sex organ in men is the testes, responsible for the production of sperm.

43. A. Vasectomy is a surgical procedure for male sterilization. During the procedure, the vas deferens are severed and then tied or sealed in such a manner that sperm are prevented from entering the seminal stream (ejaculate), thereby preventing fertilization.

44. B. *Ectopic pregnancy* is the term used to describe a pregnancy that does not occur within the uterus. Most ectopic pregnancies occur when a fertilized egg implants into the side of the fallopian tube instead of the uterus. An ectopic pregnancy can be life threatening to the woman carrying it. Although the egg can implant in such a location, the fetus will not survive.

45. D. The structure between the uterus and the vagina is the cervix.

46. A. The hormone that stimulates uterine contractions is oxytocin.

47. C. The outermost layer of the meninges is the dura mater.

48. B. The respiratory center is located in the medulla oblongata and pons.

49. D. The renal cortex is the outermost layer of each kidney.

50. A. The renal artery, renal vein, and ureter enter the kidney through the hilum.

CHAPTER 3

1. D. You should remind the team that the alarm should be activated and loud enough to be heard above other sounds in the OR to alert the staff when the ESU is activated. The sound is necessary to indicate any malfunction of the equipment.

2. D. Personnel should take special precautions when using the ESU for a patient who has a pacemaker, internal cardioverter-defibrillator, or other electrical implant.

3. A. Laminar air flow provides unidirectional positive-pressure air flow, which maintains the flow of air from inside the operating room outward. This flow of air is beneficial because it helps filter out microbes that could

compromise the sterility of the surgical area. Laminar air flow is maintained best when the operating room doors are kept closed.

4. B. The operating room is maintained at 20° to 23° C (68°–73° F). This temperature range is less hospitable to the growth of microorganisms and is comfortable for patients and personnel. (The conversion formula for Fahrenheit to Celsius is $-32 \times 5/9$. The formula for Celsius-to-Fahrenheit conversion is $\times 9/5 + 32$.)

5. D. Biomedical technologists are required to maintain the safety and operating conditions of many of the hospital's medical devices, including those used in surgery. The complexity of sophisticated devices requires technologists who have been specially trained in biomedical engineering.

6. D. The surgical suite is considered a restricted area.

7. C. Personnel must wear scrub attire, including complete head, nose, and mouth covering, in the operating room, which is a restricted area.

8. A. Decontamination is the process by which used equipment, medical devices, and surgical instrumentation are rendered safe for personnel to handle.

9. D. Disinfection is the destruction of microorganisms by heat or chemical means.

10. A. Sterilization is the process by which all microorganisms, including spores, are destroyed.

11. C. Glutaraldehyde (Cidex) is used to disinfect and sterilize surgical devices such as rigid and flexible endoscopes that require immersion. For such an instrument to be disinfected, it must be dry before being soaked or completely immersed for 20 minutes at room temperature.

12. B. The recognized minimum exposure periods for sterilization of wrapped healthcare supplies are 30 minutes at 121° C (250° F) in a gravity-displacement sterilizer or 4 minutes at 132° C (270° C) in a prevacuum sterilizer.

13. D. The Bowie-Dick test is used to detect air leaks and inadequate air removal and involves the use of folded 100% cotton surgical towels that are clean and preconditioned. A commercially available Bowie-Dick–type test sheet is placed in the center of the pack. The test pack is then placed horizontally in the front bottom section of the sterilizer rack, near the door and over the drain in an otherwise empty chamber and run at 134° C for 3.5 minutes. The test is used each day that the vacuum-type steam sterilizer is used before the first load processed.

14. A. Ultrasonic energy is routinely used by healthcare facilities to clean surgical and dental instruments before terminal sterilization. Neutral or alkaline detergents are used most commonly with ultrasonic cleaners.

15. C. Properly operated, a washer/disinfector or sterilizer is capable of killing vegetative microorganisms that can cause nosocomial infections. Be aware, however, that these products do not kill bacterial spores.

16. C. Glutaraldehyde kills *Pseudomonas spp.* and other bacteria, fungi, and viruses. It is considered a form of high-level disinfection.

17. D. Personal protective equipment consists of protective eyewear, gloves, a gown or waterproof apron, and waterproof shoe covers or boots.

18. A. The surgical technologist should inspect all electrical equipment, including cords, before surgery.

19. D. Best practices call for the surgical technologist to change a glove after recognizing that it is contaminated and informing the surgeon as well.

20. C. The best way to protect oneself from radiation during the use of a C-arm or other x-ray apparatus in the operating room is to wear a lead apron *and* thyroid shield.

CHAPTER 4

1. B. Handwashing is event related (i.e., performed before and after a specific task or event). It requires a specific method with steps that must be performed in a particular order.

2. A. Using an opened sterile single-use bottle for a second surgery is not safe because it increases the risk of carrying an infection from one patient to another.

3. C. The chain of infection requires a means of transmission. Sneezing is a means of exit for a disease to spread, not a means of transmission.

4. D. The four principles of asepsis are handwashing, clean equipment, a clean environment, and aseptic technique in a sterile field. Clean water is not one of the principles of sterile technique.

5. B. The signs of inflammation are swelling, pain, loss of function, and increased temperature. Pus formation is a sign of infection.

6. B. *Clean* means that the number of microorganisms has been reduced; *sterile* means that spore-bearing bacteria have been eliminated.

7. C. Moisture soaking through drapes, sterile or not, is called strikethrough.

8. C. The draped patient is the center of the sterile field during surgery. Other draped items and sterile personnel form the periphery of the field.

9. B. A table is considered sterile only at table height.

10. C. Sterile supplies should be opened as close to the time of surgery as possible. In reality, however, cases often are delayed or even canceled. It is not recommended that supplies be left open before a case for more than 2 hours; after 2 hours, the items should be considered contaminated, and the room should be broken down.

11. B. Sterile personnel must pass other sterile personnel back to back or front to front. Even though wraparound gowns are used in most surgical settings, the sterility of the back cannot be guaranteed because the person wearing it cannot see it.

12. A. Sterile gowns are considered sterile only in front from midchest to table level. Sterile personnel should not drop their forearms or hands below waist level or raise them above the axillary line. The axilla itself is considered nonsterile even though it is protected by a gown. This is because of the large population of bacteria in the axillary region.

13. A. One must remove and dispose of a mask immediately after leaving any restricted or semirestricted area. Even after a short time, bacterial colonization increases to a very high level on the inner surface of a mask. Masks are to be changed between surgical procedures.

14. B. The recommended practice is to remove all jewelry or completely confine it inside scrub clothes. Body piercings are considered jewelry and ideally should be confined or removed.

15. D. Aseptic technique is also known as sterile technique.

16. A. Because there are no microorganisms found in the heart, CABG is considered a clean case (class I).

17. D. The potential for bioterrorism is a reality in today's world. The Centers for Disease Control and Prevention has identified agents that may pose a risk to national security because of their (1) easy dissemination or transmission from person to person, (2) potential for high mortality and major public health impact, (3) potential to cause public panic and social disruption, and (4) requirement of special action in regard to public health preparedness. The four agents most likely to be used in acts of bioterrorism are the microorganisms that cause smallpox, plague, botulism, and tularemia.

18. A. The organisms most commonly found to be responsible for postoperative SSIs are staphylococcal, enterococcal, pseudomonal, and streptococcal species. *Staphylococcus aureus* is the most frequently identified organism.

19. B. Creutzfeldt-Jakob disease is a form of transmissible spongiform encephalopathy caused by prions.

20. A. Cidex is a trade name for glutaraldehyde, a chemical used to sterilize equipment and instruments. Glutaraldehyde treatment is considered high-level disinfection.

21. D. *Clostridium perfringens* is an anaerobic gram-positive bacterium that causes gas gangrene, cellulitis, and fasciitis.

22. C. *Helicobacter pylori*, an aerobic, gram-negative bacillus, is known to cause gastric ulcers.

23. B. The second intention heals when the wound is not sutured and gradually fills in by way of granulation.

24. D. The first intention healing that begins within minutes of an intentional and unintentional injury is known as the inflammatory phase.

25. B. Primary union wound healing takes place from side to side.

CHAPTER 5

1. B. A pulse oximeter is a digital sensor that detects oxygen saturation through the skin. The device is placed on a highly vascular area of the body (digit or earlobe) and provides continuous readings.

2. A. Neuromuscular blocking is a complex controlled process that is chemically reversed at the close of surgery or whenever necessary in the event of emergency. The drugs cause paralysis of the respiratory muscles, and mechanical ventilation is required during their use.

3. A. MAC is continuous patient monitoring provided during regional anesthesia. In addition to conducting physiological monitoring, the ACP administers sedative and anxiolytic (antianxiety) drugs as needed and manages any anesthetic or physiological emergencies.

4. D. The reversal drug for malignant hyperthermia is dantrolene.

5. A. The goal of surgical anesthesia is to allow the patient to tolerate surgery and maintain the body in a balanced physiological state called homeostasis.

6. D. Fentanyl (often sold as Sublimaze) is a narcotic.

7. C. Propofol (often sold under the brand name Diprivan) is a sedative–hypnotic.

8. B. Diazepam (Valium) is a benzodiazepine. In low doses, it produces an anxiolytic effect (relief of anxiety), and at higher doses, it causes sedation and anterograde amnesia.

9. A. Succinylcholine is a neuromuscular blocking agent. These drugs are administered to relax skeletal muscle for intubation and surgery.

10. C. Nitrous oxide is a colorless, odorless, and tasteless gas. Its mild analgesic and amnestic effects make it an excellent choice for use in conjunction with volatile anesthetics agents.

11. A. 0.9% Sodium chloride (NaCl) (isotonic) is used for fluid replacement or simple hydration. It is used in the transfusion of blood products because as it does not induce hemolysis of blood cells.

12. D. Benzodiazepines are administered at low dosages to produce an anxiolytic effect (relief of anxiety) and at higher dosages to induce sedation and anterograde amnesia. Diazepam (Valium), lorazepam (Ativan), and midazolam (Versed) are among the benzodiazepines most commonly prescribed in the surgical setting.

13. A. Metoclopramide (often sold as Reglan) is administered before surgery to reduce nausea and minimize the possibility of postoperative nausea and vomiting in at-risk patients, who include pediatric (preadolescent) patients; patients who are given opioids, barbiturates, or etomidate; and patients who are obese. Other antiemetic drugs include droperidol (Inapsine) and ondansetron (Zofran).

14. A. Common regional anesthesia techniques include spinal anesthesia (subarachnoid block), epidurals, caudals, and major peripheral nerve blocks. In epidural anesthesia, the local anesthetic is usually injected through the intervertebral spaces in the lumbar region (lumbar epidural), although it may also be injected into the cervical or thoracic region. In caudal anesthesia, the local anesthetic is also injected into the epidural space, but the approach is made through the caudal canal in the sacrum. In peripheral nerve block, the anesthetic is injected along the nerve pathway.

15. D. Nitrous oxide and halothane promote rapid induction and recovery and offer the fastest onset of induction, emergence, and recovery.

16. A. The use of nitrous oxide or opioids increases the risk of postoperative nausea and vomiting. For this reason, antiemetic drugs are given before surgery to all patients to whom nitrous oxide or opioids will be administered.

17. C. Ketamine, in large doses, can cause hallucinations and respiratory depression. The patient given ketamine needs a dark, quiet room for recovery.

18. D. The STSR should be ready to apply cricoid pressure to prevent regurgitation of stomach contents and aid the ACP in visualizing the vocal cords.

19. D. Kanamycin belongs to the aminoglycoside group, not the cephalosporin family.

20. B. Tetracycline is never administered to pediatric patients because it can permanently stain a child's teeth yellow.

21. B. Sublimaze is one of the brand names under which fentanyl citrate may be sold.

22. A. Before inflation of the double-cuff tourniquet around the extremity, an Esmarch bandage is used to induce exsanguination, enabling bloodless surgery.

23. B. The metabolic processing of a drug within the body, including absorption, distribution, biotransformation, and excretion, is known as pharmacokinetics.

24. D. In stage IV anesthesia, anesthesia is so deep that cardiovascular and respiratory function are compromised to the point of collapse as a result of depression of brain centers.

25. B. In the induction phase, a laryngeal mask airway is used to maintain the patient's airway.

CHAPTER 6

1. B. Surgical technologists are certified after successfully completing a CAAHEP- or ABHES-accredited program and passing the national Certified Surgical Technologist examination administered by the National Board of Surgical Technology and Surgical Assisting.

2. A. The primary purpose of the Association of Surgical Technologists (AST) is to ensure that surgical technologists have the knowledge and skills with which to administer patient care of the highest quality. It serves as the principal provider, in conjunction with more than 40 state organizations, of continuing education for surgical technologists. The AST also works with the Accreditation Review Council on Education in Surgical Technology and Surgical Assisting and the National Board of Surgical Technology and Surgical Assisting to set standards for education and certification; represents the profession at the state and national levels to ensure graduation from accredited programs in surgical technology; and seeks to ensure that all surgical technologists attain the Certified Surgical Technologist credential as a condition of employment.

3. B. Certification represents a permission to do something that is otherwise forbidden.

4. D. Surgical conscience is willingness to be held liable for one's own actions in providing health care to the patient—for instance, not hesitating to admit a break in aseptic technique to help prevent surgical wound infection.

5. D. According to the AST's Professional Code of Conduct, surgical technologists must represent the association or the constituent division with which that person is affiliated and shall refrain from expressing personal opinions that are contradictory to the association's positions.

6. A. Maslow's hierarchy of needs consists of five stages, which are divided into basic (or deficiency) needs (physiological, safety, love, and esteem) and growth needs (self-actualization).

7. A. Group dynamics can play a significant role in all education and learning in groups by improving interpersonal relations and communication skills. This in turn results in better group discussions, case presentations, ward rounds, skills achievement and practice sessions, and socialization, plus improved critical thinking and clarification of doubts.

8. D. Nonverbal communication is achieved, consciously or unconsciously, without talking. It may take the form of body language, facial expressions, gestures, tone of voice, touch or contact, signs, symbols, pictures, objects, and other visual aids.

9. B. Good verbal communication is the ability to present your ideas clearly through use of the spoken word and the ability to listen carefully to other people.

10. A. Erik and Joan Erikson believed that achieving a balance between autonomy and shame and doubt would lead to the development of will, the ability of a child to act with intention, within reason and limits.

CHAPTER 7

1. B. The esophagus begins at the level of C6 and passes through the neck posterior to the trachea.

2. A. The open appendectomy approach involves the use of the McBurney incision to reach the appendix, which is typically found in the right lower quadrant of the abdomen.

3. D. Gastrectomy requires clamping and ligation of the splenic vessels.

4. B. Surgical excision of the pylorus with end-to-end anastomosis of the stomach and duodenum is known as the Billroth I procedure.

5. B. Before hemorrhoidectomy, the patient is placed in the jackknife position, with the buttocks taped open laterally and secured to the sides of the operating room bed.

6. A. The liver, spleen, and pancreas are all solid (not hollow or collapsible) organs. These organs are highly vascular and control various metabolic and immune functions of the body.

7. D. The gallbladder sits in a groove on the underside of the right lobe of the liver, ending in the cystic duct. Each day the liver produces as much as 1000 mL of bile, which flows from the liver into the gallbladder for storage, where it becomes concentrated. The muscular gallbladder contracts, sending bile out into the cystic duct and then the common duct. Bile is released into the duodenum, where it works to emulsify fats, when the sphincter of Oddi in the ampulla of Vater relaxes.

8. B. In pancreaticoduodenectomy (or the Whipple procedure) the head of the pancreas, as well as the duodenum, part of the jejunum, distal third of the stomach, and lower half of the common bile duct are removed, and the biliary, pancreatic, and gastrointestinal systems are reattached.

9. B. The Hesselbach triangle is bounded by the deep epigastric vessels laterally, the inguinal ligament inferiorly, and the rectus abdominis muscle medially.

10. A. The Bartholin glands and ducts are located on each side of the lower end of the vagina. These narrow ducts open into the vaginal orifice on the inner aspects of the labia minora. The glands, which secrete mucus, may become infected or otherwise inflamed.

11. C. For an endometrial ablation, the patient is placed in the lithotomy position.

12. A. In cystocele (bladder herniation) and rectocele (rectal herniation), muscle and connective tissue weaken, resulting in prolapse against the vaginal wall.

13. A. Cerclage is a procedure in which a suture ligature is placed around the cervix to prevent spontaneous abortion.

14. B. The urethra is dilated with the use of van Buren sounds, after which the resectoscope is inserted. Resection starts with the middle and lateral lobes.

15. A. In the Marshall-Marchetti-Krantz procedure (vesicourethral suspension), the bladder neck and urethra are sutured to the cartilage of the pubic symphysis. It is performed as a means of treating urinary stress incontinence in women. A lower midline or Pfannenstiel incision into the space of Retzius is made.

16. D. Epispadias is a rare condition in which the urethral meatus is located on the top side of the penis. The defect is associated with exstrophy of the bladder and other developmental defects of the pelvis and genitourinary system.

17. C. Myringotomy is a surgical opening made in the tympanic membrane to release fluid resulting from chronic otitis media from the middle ear.

18. D. Tonsil and adenoid instruments include the Crowe-Davis gag, tonsil snare, adenoid curette, elevator, clamps, and scissors.

19. A. The lateral third of the external auditory canal is lined with glands that secrete a waxy substance called cerumen or earwax.

20. A. In total shoulder arthroplasty, artificial parts are used to replace the humeral head and glenoid capsule to restore function and relieve pain. In hemiarthroplasty, just the humeral component is replaced.

21. A. The epiphyseal plate—sometimes called the epiphysial plate, the physis, or the growth plate—is a plate of hyaline cartilage found in the metaphysis at each end of the long bones of children and adolescents. In the bones of adults, which have stopped growing, these plates are replaced by what is called the epiphyseal line.

22. B. Irregularly shaped bones that occur singly in a tendon or muscle are called sesamoid bones. The patella, or kneecap, is one example of a sesamoid bone.

23. C. The Bankart and Putti-Platt procedures are commonly used to correct chronic anterior dislocation of the shoulder. The glenoid rim is reattached to the joint capsule in the Bankart procedure; the Putti-Platt procedure involves severing the subscapularis tendon and attaching it to the glenoid.

24. D. Greenstick fractures, in which the bone bends and breaks, are common in children.

25. D. The rotator cuff, which encircles the shoulder joint, consists of four muscles: the supraspinatus, infraspinatus, teres minor, and subscapularis. The rotator cuff functions to stabilize the shoulder joint; the pectoralis major, teres major, deltoid, and latissimus dorsi muscles move the arm.

26. A. There are two ways of taking a bone graft. In the Cloward method, a special dowel cutter is used to take a plug-shaped piece of bone from the iliac crest. In the other method, the surgeon uses an osteotome and mallet to harvest slivers of bone from the iliac crest. (Both methods involve the creation of an initial incision that is deepened with the use of a monopolar electrosurgical unit and then secured with a self-retaining retractor once the bone has been exposed.) A periosteal elevator is used to strip periosteum from the crest.

27. D. A burr hole, the smallest possible access to the brain, is required in many neurosurgical procedures, including placement of a ventriculoperitoneal shunt to drain cerebrospinal fluid. When a bigger hole is needed, craniotomy may be performed. The piece of bone that is removed may be replaced after the procedure is finished, or it can be safely frozen and put back in the patient's skull after intracranial pressure has diminished.

28. C. The glossopharyngeal, trigeminal, and trochlear nerves are three of the 12 paired cranial nerves.

29. B. The Le Fort I (transverse maxillary) fracture runs horizontally through the nasal floor, the septum, and the teeth. The Le Fort II (pyramidal maxillary) fracture may be unilateral or bilateral. Generally, the nasal cavity, the hard palate, and the orbital rim are involved. Le Fort III (craniofacial dysjunction) fracture involves fractures of the nose and both zygomas. Both maxillary and mandibular fractures may be accompanied by malocclusion or even deformity of the middle of the face. Some Le Fort II fractures respond to closed reduction and intermaxillary fixation.

30. B. The TRAM (transverse rectus abdominis myocutaneous) flap procedure for breast reconstruction after mastectomy involves the use of a pedicle-based flap. It is the most commonly used component of breast reconstruction after mastectomy. The surgeon may opt to use one or both sides of the rectus muscle (the broad abdominal muscle stretching from beneath the ribs to the pubis). The superior epigastric artery and vein are carried inside the muscle pedicle to their new location. The pedicle is severed at the farthest distal point possible, a subcutaneous tunnel is made, and the muscle is pulled through the tunnel to the chest to serve as a breast. (Depending on

the size of the muscle and of the resulting breast, a small breast implant may be needed.) TRAM flap surgery also provides abdominoplasty.

31. A. Rhytidectomy, or facelift, corrects sagging of the supportive tissue of the face that is part of the aging process or may accompany some pathological conditions.

32. A. Mentoplasty is the name given to surgical augmentation of the chin.

33. D. An autograft is taken from within an individual's body and replaced in (often in another part of) that person's body.

34. A. Dupuytren disease is marked by contraction of the palmar fascia.

35. A. The extraocular muscles of the eyeball include two oblique muscles (superior and inferior) and four recti muscles (superior rectus, inferior rectus, medial rectus, lateral rectus).

36. C. Exenteration is the name given to the procedure in which the entire orbital contents, including the periosteum, are removed in the treatment of cancers of the globe or orbit.

37. D. Enucleation is the total removal of the eyeball (globe). In evisceration, the contents of the eye are removed but the outer shell of the sclera and muscle attachments are left intact.

38. D. A cataract is an opacity of the lens. Most cataracts develop as part of the aging process, but they may also be a result of genetics, injury, certain medications and diseases, or trauma.

39. A. Strabismus is a disorder in which the eye cannot focus as a result of muscle incoordination. In strabismus repair surgery, the muscles are removed and reattached in the correct locations to achieve better focus.

40. A. Phenylephrine is a mydriatic drug—that is, a medication used to dilate the pupil.

41. D. Thyroidectomy is performed in the treatment of known or suspected malignancy or hyperthyroidism. A tracheotomy set should be kept available in case bilateral cord paralysis occurs.

42. D. The three small articulating bones in the middle ear are the malleus (hammer), incus (anvil), and stapes (stirrup).

43. B. There are three paired sets of salivary glands: sublingual, submandibular, and parotid. The parotid gland, which is divided into superficial and deep portions, is the biggest of the three sets. It is found beneath the zygomatic arch in front of the mastoid process and behind the ramus of the mandible. Stensen's duct, also known as the parotid duct, tunnels through the buccal fat pad and the buccinator muscle and opens into the oral cavity opposite the crown of the upper second molar.

44. B. The incision is made through the pars plana layer, one of the three layers of the eye, located near the where the iris and sclera join.

45. C. The intraocular gases that are mixed with sterile air and used to flatten a detached retina to keep it attached during the healing process are sulfur hexafluoride (SF6), perfluoroethane (C2F6), and perfluoropropane (C3F8). Nitrous oxide is not used in this way.

46. A. Heterotopic transplantation, in which the patient's diseased heart is left in place to support a newly transplanted donor heart, is also known as piggyback transplantation.

47. B. The brachial nerve does not innervate the hand.

48. D. Blood moves in veins when skeletal muscle contracts.

49. B. The tunica media is made up of smooth muscle.

50. A. PTFE (polytetrafluoroethylene) is chosen for below-the-knee graft procedures.

ANSWER KEY FOR PRINT PRACTICE EXAM

1. D. Mannitol is an osmotic diuretic that reduces intracranial pressure.
   CST Exam Topic: III. Basic Science; C. Surgical Pharmacology

2. D. The Finochietto retractor is a self-retaining chest retractor.
   CST Exam Topic: I. Peri-Operative Care; A. Pre-Operative Preparation

3. D. Glycine is the medium of choice here; non-electrolytic solutions are used for distention during cystoscopy procedures.
   CST Exam Topic: III. Basic Science; C. Surgical Pharmacology

4. C. Cranial nerve VII, the facial nerve, is at risk for damage during rhytidectomy.
   CST Exam Topic: III. Basic Science; A. Anatomy and Physiology

5. D. In surgical repair of hip fracture, the patient is placed in the supine position with the affected leg placed in a traction boot on the fracture table.
   CST Exam Topic: I. Peri-Operative Care; A. Pre-Operative Preparation

6. D. Creutzfeldt-Jakob disease is caused by prions. Transmission of these prions on surgical instruments, particularly those used during neurosurgical procedures, is possible. Prions are very resistant to chemical and physical sterilization methods such as pressurized steam, ethylene oxide, and dry heat. The World Health Organization's Infection Control Guidelines for Transmissible Spongiform Encephalopathies recommend the use of single-use disposable instruments and the destruction of all reusable instruments when prion exposure is a possibility.
   CST Exam Topic: III. Basic Science; B. Microbiology

7. C. Infection with *Clostridium perfringens*, a common cause of gas gangrene, is more likely in patients with poor circulation, such as those with diabetes.
   CST Exam Topic: III. Basic Science; B. Microbiology

8. C. Standard precautions were defined by the Centers for Disease Control and Prevention in 1996 to protect healthcare workers against blood and *all* body fluids, secretions, and excretions except sweat. Whether or not they contain visible blood, all body fluids should be treated as if they are potentially infectious, and the skin and mucous membranes of healthcare workers should be protected from these fluids to reduce the risk of transmission of microorganisms. Gloves should be worn at all times by anyone working with body fluids.
   CST Exam Topic: III. Basic Science; B. Microbiology

9. D. Hepatitis B virus (HBV) is the only one of these microorganisms that can be transmitted through a needlestick.
   CST Exam Topic: III. Basic Science; B. Microbiology

10. B. Hypaque is a contract medium used in radiographic procedures. The other three options are types of dyes.
    CST Exam Topic: III. Basic Science; C. Surgical Pharmacology

11. C. Dantrolene sodium (Dantrium) is the pharmacologic agent administered specifically for the direct treatment of malignant hyperthermic (MH) crisis. Furosemide (Lasix), a loop diuretic, is also administered during an MH crisis.
    CST Exam Topic: III. Basic Science; C. Surgical Pharmacology

12. C. A patient undergoing pilonidal cystectomy is placed in the prone position because these cysts occur in the sacral area.
    CST Exam Topic: I. Peri-Operative Care; A. Pre-Operative Preparation

13. B. The CST should anticipate that the surgeon performing an appendectomy will use atraumatic forceps (e.g., Babcock forceps) to avoid perforation or spillage of the appendix.
    CST Exam Topic: I. Peri-Operative Care; B. Intra-Operative Procedures

14. D. The surgeon is responsible for managing a fractured extremity during the transfer of a patient to the operating room table.
    CST Exam Topic: I. Peri-Operative Care; A. Pre-Operative Preparation

15. D. The best choice of action would be to break down the entire setup and start fresh before beginning the surgical procedure.
    CST Exam Topic: I. Peri-Operative Care; A. Pre-Operative Preparation

16. C. The thigh is the optimal placement site for the grounding pad.
    CST Exam Topic: I. Peri-Operative Care; A. Pre-Operative Preparation

17. D. Whenever there is a break in sterile technique, the individual who notices the break must notify the individual who has committed the break in technique, after which a recovery action plan can be implemented.
    CST Exam Topic: I. Peri-Operative Care; B. Intra-Operative Procedures

18. D. For laparoscopic assisted vaginal hysterectomy, the patient is placed in the lithotomy position.
    CST Exam Topic: I. Peri-Operative Care; A. Pre-Operative Preparation

19. A. Before incision, the best choice of action is to break down the setup, reprep, and redrape.
    CST Exam Topic: I. Peri-Operative Care; A. Pre-Operative Preparation

20. D. A high degree of static electricity is directly correlated with high humidity.
    CST Exam Topic: I. Peri-Operative Care; A. Pre-Operative Preparation

21. D. A C-section procedure requires an additional count because it involves entry into the uterus (i.e., an extra cavity).
    CST Exam Topic: I. Peri-Operative Care; B. Intra-Operative Procedures

22. D. Monopolar cautery is the only one of the choices that involves heat (thermal).
    CST Exam Topic: II. Additional Duties; B. Equipment Sterilization and Maintenance

23. D. Whenever instrumentation is added to the sterile field, the new instruments must be added to the count.
    CST Exam Topic: I. Peri-Operative Care; B. Intra-Operative Procedures

24. D. The patellar tendon is routinely used as a graft in anterior cruciate ligament reconstruction. An autograft is one that is taken from the patient's own tissue.
    CST Exam Topic: I. Peri-Operative Care; B. Intra-Operative Procedures

25. D. The best choice of action would be to notify the surgeon and stop the wound closure.
    CST Exam Topic: I. Peri-Operative Care; B. Intra-Operative Procedures

26. C. As a means of facilitating decontamination and disinfection, all instrumentation should be unlocked and disassembled. NaCl solution should never be used to clean instrumentation.
    CST Exam Topic: II. Additional Duties; B. Equipment Sterilization and Maintenance

27. C. In retention sutures, a secondary suture line is used to prevent dehiscence.
    CST Exam Topic: I. Peri-Operative Care; B. Intra-Operative Procedures

28. A. Autoclave tape is a chemical indicator that confirms exposure to the sterilization process.
    CST Exam Topic: II. Additional Duties; B. Equipment Sterilization and Maintenance

29. A. *Bacillus stearothermophilus* is the microorganism used in biological indicators to challenge and validate the steam sterilization process.
    CST Exam Topic: II. Additional Duties; B. Equipment Sterilization and Maintenance

30. D. Intact skin is the body's first line of defense against infection. For this reason, burn victims are at risk for infection.
    CST Exam Topic: III. Basic Science; B. Microbiology

31. A. Low hemoglobin is a cause for concern. The normal hemoglobin range in men is 13.5 to 18 g/dL; in women, it is 11.5 to 15.5 g/dL.
    CST Exam Topic: I. Peri-Operative Care; A. Pre-Operative Preparation

32. D. The Sellick maneuver is used to occlude the esophagus and prevent aspiration.
    CST Exam Topic: I. Peri-Operative Care; A. Pre-Operative Preparation

33. D. The surgeon, not the CST, is responsible for obtaining the informed consent.
    CST Exam Topic: I. Peri-Operative Care; A. Pre-Operative Preparation

34. A. The surgeon is responsible for obtaining informed consent, so a nurse's obtaining consent would invalidate the consent.
    CST Exam Topic: I. Peri-Operative Care; A. Pre-Operative Preparation

35. C. Class II wound healing involves granulation.
    CST Exam Topic: III. Basic Science; B. Microbiology

36. B. Early ambulation promotes good wound healing.
    CST Exam Topic: I. Peri-Operative Care; C. Post-Operative Procedures

37. D. In the healthcare setting, *Res ipsa loquitur* (Latin for "The thing speaks for itself") refers to an act so obviously below the standard of practice that negligence is assumed.
    CST Exam Topic: II. Additional Duties; A. Administrative and Personnel

38. D. Malpractice includes performing a task outside the scope of one's job description.
    CST Exam Topic: II. Additional Duties; A. Administrative and Personnel

39. C. Calling in sick does not require the filing of an incident report.
    CST Exam Topic: II. Additional Duties; A. Administrative and Personnel

40. C. Radiological procedures require the use of lead aprons and thyroid shields for protection against radiation.
    CST Exam Topic: I. Peri-Operative Care; A. Pre-Operative Preparation

41. D. Gowning and gloving should be conducted at either the Mayo stand or a separate table.
    CST Exam Topic: I. Peri-Operative Care; A. Pre-Operative Preparation

42. C. Laser safety glasses are required for all individuals who must work in proximity to a laser beam.
    CST Exam Topic: I. Peri-Operative Care; A. Pre-Operative Preparation

43. C. A CST who has scrubbed for a surgical procedure may not leave during the procedure until relieved by another staff member; leaving without being relieved constitutes abandonment of the patient.
    CST Exam Topic: II. Additional Duties; A. Administrative and Personnel

44. B. Glutaraldehyde, commonly sold under the brand name Cidex, is a high-level disinfectant. It is recognized as one of the best overall disinfectants and liquid sterilants on the market. A minimum exposure of 20 minutes at room temperature is required for high-level disinfection. An item must be immersed in glutaraldehyde for at least 10 hours to be rendered sterile.
    CST Exam Topic: II. Additional Duties; B. Equipment Sterilization and Maintenance

45. C. Colposcopy is an unsterile procedure that is usually performed in a physician's office.
    CST Exam Topic: I. Peri-Operative Care; B. Intra-Operative Procedures

46. C. Gowned and gloved individuals within the sterile field must pass each other facing front to front (sterile to sterile) or back to back (unsterile to unsterile).
    CST Exam Topic: I. Peri-Operative Care; B. Intra-Operative Procedures

47. D. A sterile field is created 12 to 18 inches from any unsterile furniture or walls.
    CST Exam Topic: I. Peri-Operative Care; A. Pre-Operative Preparation

48. C. A sterile field must be monitored at all times to ensure sterility; when sterility is in doubt, the field must be considered nonsterile.
    CST Exam Topic: I. Peri-Operative Care; A. Pre-Operative Preparation

49. B. The CST has altered the degree of sterility. The only time sitting is allowed in the sterile field is if the entire procedure will be performed with the staff in the seated position.
    CST Exam Topic: I. Peri-Operative Care; A. Pre-Operative Preparation

50. D. Implants are never allowed to be flashed; they must be sterilized and held for 24 hours to ensure that the biological run with the implant load is negative.
    CST Exam Topic: II. Additional Duties; B. Equipment Sterilization and Maintenance

51. C. The surgeon's informing the patient of the risks and benefits of the procedure is essential to obtaining valid informed consent.
    CST Exam Topic: I. Peri-Operative Care; A. Pre-Operative Preparation

52. C. When a patient is placed in the lithotomy position, both legs are raised simultaneously and placed in stirrups.
    CST Exam Topic: I. Peri-Operative Care; A. Pre-Operative Preparation

53. D. DuraPrep and all one-step prepping solutions should be allowed adequate drying time prior to incision.
    CST Exam Topic: I. Peri-Operative Care; A. Pre-Operative Preparation

54. D. Specimens containing stones or teeth should be sent to pathology in a dry container without any solution.
    CST Exam Topic: I. Peri-Operative Care; B. Intra-Operative Procedures

55. D. Pediatric preoperative preparation should include having temperature-regulation devices available for the procedure.
    CST Exam Topic: I. Peri-Operative Care; A. Pre-Operative Preparation

56. D. Increased CO_2 level (not increased), muscle rigidity, unexplained tachycardia, and increased temperature are all symptoms of malignant hyperthermic crisis.
    CST Exam Topic: I. Peri-Operative Care; B. Intra-Operative Procedures

57. B. Pressure dressings and drains are used to eliminate dead space.
    CST Exam Topic: I. Peri-Operative Care; C. Post-Operative Procedures

58. D. Class IV wound classification is applied to patients who are already infected at the start of a procedure.
    CST Exam Topic: III. Basic Science; B. Microbiology

59. B. The T-tube is primarily used for drainage within the biliary system and the common bile duct for passage of stones.
    CST Exam Topic: I. Peri-Operative Care; B. Intra-Operative Procedures

60. D. The Salem sump tube is a double-lumen gastric drainage tube that is inserted orally to draw out fluid or gas.
    CST Exam Topic: I. Peri-Operative Care; B. Intra-Operative Procedures

61. A. Stones are sent to pathology for analysis in a dry specimen container.
    CST Exam Topic: I. Peri-Operative Care; B. Intra-Operative Procedures

62. D. Removal of the bladder and urinary diversion procedures require reconstruction of a new reservoir for urine output. This is created from the ileum.
    CST Exam Topic: I. Peri-Operative Care; B. Intra-Operative Procedures

63. D. Silk suture is contraindicated in the genitourinary and biliary systems because it promotes stone formation.
    CST Exam Topic: I. Peri-Operative Care; B. Intra-Operative Procedures

64. D. Strabismus surgery involves the extrinsic eye muscles, so instrumentation includes the caliper for accurate measurement and a muscle hook for retraction.
    CST Exam Topic: I. Peri-Operative Care; B. Intra-Operative Procedures

65. D. Split-thickness skin grafting involves the use of a dermatome, graft expansion device, mineral oil, and cotton balls.
    CST Exam Topic: I. Peri-Operative Care; B. Intra-Operative Procedures

66. C. Drill, measure, tap, and screw are the correct steps for screw fixation placement.
    CST Exam Topic: I. Peri-Operative Care; B. Intra-Operative Procedures

67. D. A patient undergoing total hip arthroplasty would be positioned laterally, with the affected extremity superior.
    CST Exam Topic: I. Peri-Operative Care; A. Pre-Operative Preparation

68. B. Triple arthrodesis fusion involves the talus, navicular, and calcaneus. The ilium is not located in the lower extremity.
    CST Exam Topic: III. Basic Science; A. Anatomy and Physiology

69. D. The Javid shunt is essential to maintaining oxygenated blood flow to the brain during carotid endarterectomy.
    CST Exam Topic: I. Peri-Operative Care; B. Intra-Operative Procedures

70. D. Papaverine is used to prevent vasospasm during vascular procedures.
   CST Exam Topic: III. Basic Science; C. Surgical Pharmacology

71. D. Active drains have suction, and the Hemovac drain is ideal for this procedure.
   CST Exam Topic: I. Peri-Operative Care; A. Pre-Operative Preparation

72. C. Bowel isolation technique is used to isolate surgical instrumentation that has come in contact with *Escherichia coli.*
   CST Exam Topic: I. Peri-Operative Care; B. Intra-Operative Procedures

73. D. Anatomically, the splenic flexure of the large intestine involves the transverse colon and the descending colon.
   CST Exam Topic: III. Basic Science; A. Anatomy and Physiology

74. D. To prevent fire, the light source should be placed on standby when the scope is outside the abdomen.
   CST Exam Topic: I. Peri-Operative Care; B. Intra-Operative Procedures

75. A. The Hasson technique does not require the use of a Veress needle.
   CST Exam Topic: I. Peri-Operative Care; B. Intra-Operative Procedures

76. C. An argon laser is used in retinal detachment repair.
   CST Exam Topic: I. Peri-Operative Care; A. Pre-Operative Preparation

77. D. Westcott scissors are used in ophthalmic procedures.
   CST Exam Topic: I. Peri-Operative Care; A. Pre-Operative Preparation

78. B. Anterior pelvic exenteration involves removal of the bladder, fallopian tubes, ovaries, and uterus to treat carcinoma.
   CST Exam Topic: I. Peri-Operative Care; B. Intra-Operative Procedures

79. C. Gibson and flank incisions give the surgical team access to the kidney.
   CST Exam Topic: I. Peri-Operative Care; B. Intra-Operative Procedures

80. D. A three-way Foley catheter is inserted after surgery to aid in hemostasis.
   CST Exam Topic: I. Peri-Operative Care; B. Intra-Operative Procedures

81. B. The suprapubic approach involves the use of the Pfannenstiel incision to gain entry to the bladder and prostate.
   CST Exam Topic: I. Peri-Operative Care; B. Intra-Operative Procedures

82. C. The Bankart procedure involves the shoulder; the labrum is the cartilage that surrounds the glenoid of the shoulder.
   CST Exam Topic: III. Basic Science; A. Anatomy and Physiology

83. C. The patellar tendon is the most commonly used source of autograft for the anterior cruciate ligament procedure.
   CST Exam Topic: III. Basic Science; A. Anatomy and Physiology

84. C. The most common diagnosis associated with arthroplasty is osteoarthritis.
   CST Exam Topic: I. Peri-Operative Care; A. Pre-Operative Preparation

85. C. The circle of Willis is the most likely anatomical site of a cerebral aneurysm.
   CST Exam Topic: III. Basic Science; A. Anatomy and Physiology

86. A. The tip of the mastoid process is located in close proximity to the facial nerve.
   CST Exam Topic: III. Basic Science; A. Anatomy and Physiology

87. B. Cerebral aneurysm clips can never be reused.
   CST Exam Topic: I. Peri-Operative Care; B. Intra-Operative Procedures

88. C. The proximal end of the shunt is placed in the ventricle to aid drainage of cerebrospinal fluid.
   CST Exam Topic: I. Peri-Operative Care; B. Intra-Operative Procedures

89. C. The iliac crest is the preferred site for autograft bone harvesting.
   CST Exam Topic: III. Basic Science; A. Anatomy and Physiology

90. C. The glenoid is anatomical bone located within the shoulder joint.
   CST Exam Topic: III. Basic Science; A. Anatomy and Physiology

91. C. The correct sequence of draping for a patient in lithotomy position is the under-buttock drape, leggings, and an abdominal sheet.
   CST Exam Topic: I. Peri-Operative Care; A. Pre-Operative Preparation

92. C. The best choice is to prep the harvesting area first and the wound site second, clean to dirty, using two individual prep sets.
   CST Exam Topic: I. Peri-Operative Care; A. Pre-Operative Preparation

93. B. The best choice of action would be to cover the contaminated area and isolate because the incision has already been made and Marco is in the middle of the procedure. He may inform the surgeon but may not dictate a medication order.
   CST Exam Topic: I. Peri-Operative Care; A. Pre-Operative Preparation

94. A. The Trendelenburg position allows the pelvic contents to displace cephalad and permits greater visibility and accessibility by the surgical team.
   CST Exam Topic: I. Peri-Operative Care; A. Pre-Operative Preparation

95. D. The beanbag positioner is specifically used for patients who are placed in the lateral position.
   CST Exam Topic: I. Peri-Operative Care; A. Pre-Operative Preparation

96. D. The best choice of action is to break down the setup and ensure that the fly is removed from operating room to prevent contamination.
   CST Exam Topic: I. Peri-Operative Care; A. Pre-Operative Preparation

97. D. Evisceration is the separation of a surgical wound and spillage of viscera after the surgery.
   CST Exam Topic: I. Peri-Operative Care; C. Post-Operative Procedures

98. A. Allowing separation of wound layers promotes dead space.
   CST Exam Topic: I. Peri-Operative Care; C. Post-Operative Procedures

99. D. Secondary intention wound healing is associated with tissue granulation.
   CST Exam Topic: I. Peri-Operative Care; C. Post-Operative Procedures

100. C. Sterile drapes, after they have been placed, may not be moved.
   CST Exam Topic: I. Peri-Operative Care; A. Pre-Operative Preparation

101. D. Dressing sponges are not counted and should not be opened onto the sterile field until the final count is completed.
   CST Exam Topic: I. Peri-Operative Care; A. Pre-Operative Preparation

102. C. The Gerota fascia surrounds and protects the kidney.
   CST Exam Topic: III. Basic Science; A. Anatomy and Physiology

103. B. Any white blood cell count greater than 10,000/mm³ indicates the presence of infection.
   CST Exam Topic: III. Basic Science; B. Microbiology

104. B. Negligence is the commission (or omission) of some act that a reasonable or prudent person would not commit (or neglect to commit) under the same conditions.
   CST Exam Topic: II. Additional Duties; A. Administrative and Personnel

105. C. Glutaraldehyde is a liquid disinfectant and sterilizing agent that is often sold under the brand name Cidex. The fumes can be irritating to the eyes and mucous membranes. When not in use, glutaraldehyde must be kept in a covered container.
   CST Exam Topic: II. Additional Duties; B. Equipment Sterilization and Maintenance

106. C. Nonsterile surgical team members must maintain a distance of 12 to 18 inches from the sterile field, so a distance of 6 inches would break sterility.
   CST Exam Topic: I. Peri-Operative Care; A. Pre-Operative Preparation

107. D. Sharps containers must be handled carefully.
   CST Exam Topic: I. Peri-Operative Care; A. Pre-Operative Preparation

108. A. Gowning off a separate table or Mayo stand is acceptable sterile technique.
   CST Exam Topic: I. Peri-Operative Care; A. Pre-Operative Preparation

109. C. Thrombin may never be injected.
   CST Exam Topic: III. Basic Science; C. Surgical Pharmacology

110. D. The universal donor is type O, and the universal recipient type is AB.
   CST Exam Topic: III. Basic Science; B. Microbiology

111. A. Dantrolene is used specifically to treat malignant hyperthermia, and furosemide (Lasix) is a diuretic.
   CST Exam Topic: III. Basic Science; C. Surgical Pharmacology

112. C. Dexamethasone (Decadron) is a steroid used to reduce inflammation.
   CST Exam Topic: III. Basic Science; C. Surgical Pharmacology

113. D. Papaverine is a vasodilator used to prevent vasospasm.
   CST Exam Topic: III. Basic Science; C. Surgical Pharmacology

114. D. The Sellick maneuver is used to prevent aspiration.
   CST Exam Topic: I. Peri-Operative Care; A. Pre-Operative Preparation

115. B. Double-armed polypropylene is used for vascular anastomosis.
   CST Exam Topic: I. Peri-Operative Care; A. Pre-Operative Preparation

116. D. The sterile field must be monitored and therefore may never be left alone.
   CST Exam Topic: I. Peri-Operative Care; A. Pre-Operative Preparation

117. D. The circulator is unsterile and may not enter the sterile field.
   CST Exam Topic: I. Peri-Operative Care; A. Pre-Operative Preparation

118. D. The semirestricted area requires scrubs, hat, and booties; the restricted area requires scrubs, hat, booties, and mask.
   CST Exam Topic: I. Peri-Operative Care; A. Pre-Operative Preparation

119. D. Pulse lavage is used intraoperatively before bone cement application to prevent the formation of microemboli.
   CST Exam Topic: I. Peri-Operative Care; B. Intra-Operative Procedures

120. B. The Duval clamp is used to grasp lung tissue.
   CST Exam Topic: I. Peri-Operative Care; B. Intra-Operative Procedures

121. D. The Hesselbach triangle is the area bounded by the rectus abdominis muscle, the inguinal ligament, and the inferior epigastric vessels, the anatomy associated with direct inguinal hernia.
   CST Exam Topic: III. Basic Science; A. Anatomy and Physiology

122. C. A Penrose drain is used to retract the spermatic cord during hernia repair.
   CST Exam Topic: I. Peri-Operative Care; B. Intra-Operative Procedures

123. C. Desired/Available × Quantity
   D = 500 mg A = 250 mg × 1 mg
   500 mg/250 mg × 1 = 500 ÷ 250 = 2 mL
   CST Exam Topic: III. Basic Science; C. Surgical Pharmacology

124. D. The Billroth procedure involves the stomach.
   CST Exam Topic: III. Basic Science; A. Anatomy and Physiology

125. D. Cranial nerve X is the vagus nerve.
CST Exam Topic: III. Basic Science; A. Anatomy and Physiology

126. C. Linear cutters are used to transect and ligate the stump of the appendix.
CST Exam Topic: I. Peri-Operative Care; B. Intra-Operative Procedures

127. D. Bowel isolation technique is used to isolate instrumentation that has come in contact with *Escherichia coli.* To prevent the spread of the microorganism, these instruments are isolated and not used on healthy tissue.
CST Exam Topic: I. Peri-Operative Care; B. Intra-Operative Procedures

128. C. The left ventricle pumps oxygenated (not deoxygenated) blood into the aorta and systemic circulation.
CST Exam Topic: III. Basic Science; A. Anatomy and Physiology

129. C. The Harmonic scalpel cuts and cauterizes tissue by means of ultrasonic energy.
CST Exam Topic: I. Peri-Operative Care; B. Intra-Operative Procedures

130. D. Immediate use steam sterilization (flash sterilization) standards require powered instruments and instruments with lumens to be run for at least 10 minutes.
CST Exam Topic: II. Additional Duties; B. Equipment Sterilization and Maintenance

131. D. The surgeon is responsible for explaining the risks and benefits of the procedure and obtaining informed consent.
CST Exam Topic: I. Peri-Operative Care; A. Pre-Operative Preparation

132. D. Colporrhaphy is performed with the patient in the lithotomy position.
CST Exam Topic: I. Peri-Operative Care; B. Intra-Operative Procedures

133. D. Sterile Doppler ultrasonography is used to check for pulses in and patency within arteries during vascular procedures.
CST Exam Topic: I. Peri-Operative Care; B. Intra-Operative Procedures

134. C. D/A × Q =
Desired 60 mg/available 30 mg per mL/Quantity 1 mL
2 mL
CST Exam Topic: III. Basic Science; C. Surgical Pharmacology

135. A. Gross spillage is categorized as class III. In class IV, the patient presents with an infection or an open wound that is 4 hours old or older.
CST Exam Topic: I. Peri-Operative Care; B. Intra-Operative Procedures

136. C. The T-tube is always associated with the common bile duct.
CST Exam Topic: I. Peri-Operative Care; A. Pre-Operative Preparation

137. D. The muscle layer of the uterus is the myometrium.
CST Exam Topic: III. Basic Science; A. Anatomy and Physiology

138. C. During cranial procedures, the temperature of irrigation solution should be below 120° F; irrigation fluid that is too cold can contribute to hypothermia.
CST Exam Topic: I. Peri-Operative Care; B. Intra-Operative Procedures

139. C. Pituitary tumors are the pathology treated with transsphenoidal hypophysectomy.
CST Exam Topic: I. Peri-Operative Care; B. Intra-Operative Procedures

140. D. During thyroidectomy, it is a recognized practice to have a tracheostomy tray in the room and on standby.
CST Exam Topic: I. Peri-Operative Care; B. Intra-Operative Procedures

141. D. During intramedullary rodding, the greater trochanter is used as a landmark to gain entry to the femoral canal.
CST Exam Topic: I. Peri-Operative Care; B. Intra-Operative Procedures

142. C. A Colle fracture involves the distal radius.
CST Exam Topic: III. Basic Science; A. Anatomy and Physiology

143. C. The Marshall-Marchetti-Krantz procedure is an open procedure performed to correct stress incontinence in female patients.
CST Exam Topic: I. Peri-Operative Care; B. Intra-Operative Procedures

144. C. Aneurysm clips are used in neuroaneurysm procedures.
CST Exam Topic: I. Peri-Operative Care; B. Intra-Operative Procedures

145. D. Varicocelectomy is performed to ligate enlarged veins in the scrotum, sometimes as a means of improving spermatogenesis.
CST Exam Topic: I. Peri-Operative Care; B. Intra-Operative Procedures

146. A. The pairing of radial artery and cephalic vein is the best choice for arteriovenous fistula creation.
CST Exam Topic: I. Peri-Operative Care; B. Intra-Operative Procedures

147. D. The Satinsky clamp is a large vascular clamp that is often used to clamp large blood vessels.
CST Exam Topic: I. Peri-Operative Care; B. Intra-Operative Procedures

148. C. Cranial nerve VII is the facial nerve, located in close proximity to the incision in rhytidectomy.
CST Exam Topic: III. Basic Science; A. Anatomy and Physiology

149. D. Mentoplasty involves the chin, so a head and neck drape is needed.
CST Exam Topic: III. Basic Science; A. Anatomy and Physiology

150. D. Sensorineural deafness is associated with cranial nerve VIII cranial (vestibulocochlear).
CST Exam Topic: III. Basic Science; A. Anatomy and Physiology

151. D. The ethmoid sinuses are located between the eyes.
CST Exam Topic: III. Basic Science; A. Anatomy and Physiology

152. D. The trephine is used to cut out diseased cornea and cut donor cornea to fit as a graft.
CST Exam Topic: I. Peri-Operative Care; B. Intra-Operative Procedures

153. A. During intracapsular cataract extraction, an incision is made, and the diseased lens is removed en bloc. This technique is an older approach to cataract surgery that does not involve use of the phaco machine.
CST Exam Topic: I. Peri-Operative Care; B. Intra-Operative Procedures

154. C. The dacryocystorhinostomy procedure is performed to treat an occluded nasolacrimal sac.
CST Exam Topic: I. Peri-Operative Care; B. Intra-Operative Procedures

155. D. Heager dilators are obstetric/gynecologic instrumentation used to dilate the cervix.
CST Exam Topic: I. Peri-Operative Care; B. Intra-Operative Procedures

156. C. The Ellik evacuator is used to remove prostatic chips from the bladder during the cysto procedure.
CST Exam Topic: I. Peri-Operative Care; B. Intra-Operative Procedures

157. B. Malignancy of the sigmoid colon is the pathology associated with abdominal perineal resection. An end-to-end stapling device is used for anastomosis of the nonmalignant tissue of the descending colon and rectum.
CST Exam Topic: I. Peri-Operative Care; B. Intra-Operative Procedures

158. D. The Adson-Beckman retractor is a self-retaining retractor with articulating arms.
CST Exam Topic: I. Peri-Operative Care; A. Pre-Operative Preparation

159. D. The fibula is the preferred choice for autograft in this procedure.
CST Exam Topic: III. Basic Science; A. Anatomy and Physiology

160. C. The priority in tracheostomy procedures is ensuring patency of the tracheostomy balloon.
CST Exam Topic: I. Peri-Operative Care; A. Pre-Operative Preparation

161. D. Lugol solution is an iodine-based solution used in the Schiller test as a staining agent to isolate abnormal tissue.
CST Exam Topic: I. Peri-Operative Care; A. Pre-Operative Preparation

162. C. The prep for vaginal procedures begins at the pubic area and moves outward.
CST Exam Topic: I. Peri-Operative Care; A. Pre-Operative Preparation

163. B. The endobag is used to contain the specimen and prevent spillage of bile. Spillage could result in postoperative infection and would change the wound classification.
CST Exam Topic: I. Peri-Operative Care; A. Pre-Operative Preparation

164. C. The patient will have a weakened immune system because the spleen is the largest organ of the immune system.
CST Exam Topic: III. Basic Science; B. Microbiology

165. D. In vasovasotomy, the patient is placed in the supine position, not the lithotomy position.
CST Exam Topic: I. Peri-Operative Care; A. Pre-Operative Preparation

166. A. A gram-positive bacterium stains blue; a gram-negative bacterium stains pink.
CST Exam Topic: III. Basic Science; B. Microbiology

167. D. Ray-Tec sponges are counted items and should never be removed from the operating room.
CST Exam Topic: I. Peri-Operative Care; A. Pre-Operative Preparation

168. C. The Lahey thyroid clamp is a grasping instrument that would perforate the intestine if used in an intestinal procedure.
CST Exam Topic: I. Peri-Operative Care; A. Pre-Operative Preparation

169. C. A throat pack should be included in the count.
CST Exam Topic: I. Peri-Operative Care; B. Intra-Operative Procedures

170. D. The mesh graft device is used to expand the size of a harvested skin autograft.
CST Exam Topic: I. Peri-Operative Care; A. Pre-Operative Preparation

171. B. The thigh is generally the best site for grounding pad placement for monopolar cautery.
CST Exam Topic: I. Peri-Operative Care; A. Pre-Operative Preparation

172. D. Open reduction and internal fixation of a hip fracture does not involve the use of a tourniquet.
CST Exam Topic: I. Peri-Operative Care; A. Pre-Operative Preparation

173. D. Preventing blood clots from entering the pulmonary system is the goal of the procedure.
CST Exam Topic: I. Peri-Operative Care; A. Pre-Operative Preparation

174. C. Fogarty catheters are used to remove emboli from arteries and veins.
CST Exam Topic: I. Peri-Operative Care; A. Pre-Operative Preparation

175. B. Protamine sulfate is the antagonist of heparin.
CST Exam Topic: III. Basic Science; C. Surgical Pharmacology

A

Abandonment, 86
Abbreviations, medical, 4, 5t
Abdomen
 hernias, 15f
 quadrants, 12, 13f
 regions, 12, 13f
Abdominal aortic aneurysm repair, 27t, 33
Abdominal contents surgeries, 94–97
 gynecologic, 103–105
Abdominal wall, surgeries for, 92–94, 93f
Abdominoplasty, 136
Abducens nerve, 27, 29f
Accessory nerve, 28, 29f
Accreditation Review Council on Education in
 Surgical Technology and Surgical Assisting
 (ARC-STSA), 83
Accrediting Bureau of Health Education Schools
 (ABHES), 83
Achilles tendon, repair of, 117b
Acid-fast staining, 61, 62f
Acinebacter sp., 61
Adenoidectomy, 21t, 100, 101b
Adenoids, 25
Adrenal glands, 21
Adrenalectomy, 19t
Adrenocorticotrophic hormone (ACTH), 23
Adson tissue forceps, 41t–49t
Aeger primo, 86
Aerobic gram-negative bacteria, 61
Aerobic gram-positive bacteria, 60
Affidavit, 87
Allen intestinal clamps, 41t–49t
Allis forceps, 41t–49t
Alternating current (AC), definition of, 50t
American College of Surgeons (ACS), 83
Amikacin, 76
Amikin. *see* Amikacin
Aminoglycosides, 76
Aminopenicillins, 77
Amoxicillin, 77
Ampicillin, 77
Amputation, procedures for, 113–117
Anaerobic gram-negative bacteria, 61
Anaerobic gram-positive bacteria, 60
Analgesics
 as postoperative drug, 78
 as preoperative drug, 75, 75f
Anastomoses, 140b, 140
Anatomy, physiology and, 8–37, 9f, 35f
Ancef. *see* Cefazolin
Anesthesia
 local, 78
 phases of, 73, 74t
 regional, 78
 for same-day surgery, 78
Aneurysm of ascending aorta, repair of, 11–12,
 11f, 12t
Annuloplasty, mitral ring, 122

Anspor. *see* Cefradine
Antacids, 75
Anterior cruciate ligament (ACL) reconstruction,
 arthroscopic, 113b
Anterior pituitary gland, 23
Antibiotics, 76–77, 76f
 intravenous, 78–79
Anticholinergics, 75–76
Antiemetic/gastrointestinal prokinetics, 75
Antisialagogue effect, 75
Anus
 anatomical structures of, 18f
 procedures in, 18
Aortic aneurysm repair, abdominal, 27t, 33
Aortic valve replacement, 10t, 10–11
Appendectomy, 23t, 27
Argon beam, 40
Army/Navy retractors, 41t–49t
Arteries, 10t–31t, 31f
 veins *versus*, 137t, 139f
Arteriography, 138
Arteriovenous fistula, 27t, 32–33, 32f, 140b
Arteriovenous shunt, 27t, 32–33, 32f
Arteriovenous sinus. *see* Arteriovenous fistula
Arthroplasty, procedures for, 115–116
Arthroscopy, procedures for, 111–113
Articulation, definition of, 51t
Ascending aorta, aneurysm of, repair of, 11–12,
 11f, 12t
Association of Perioperative Nurses, 83
Association of Surgical Technologists (AST), 83
 code of ethics of, 88b
Atropine, 75
Attorney, durable power of, for health care, 87
Autonomy *versus* shame and doubt, on Erikson's
 psychosocial stages, 85
Auvard weighted speculums, 41t–49t
Azithromycin, 77

B

Babcock forceps, 41t–49t
Bacampicillin, 77
Bacillus anthracis, 60
Bacillus subtilis, 55
Bacteremia, 60
Bacteria, characteristics of, 59–61
Bactericidal penicillins, 77
Bacteroides fragilis, 61
Bakes dilators, 41t–49t
Balfour retractors, 41t–49t
Bankart procedure, 117f
Baron suction tip, 41t–49t
Bartholin abscess, 105f
Bartholin gland, marsupialization of, 105, 106b
Bartonella sp., 61
Beach chair-style shoulder positioner, 114f
Benzodiazepines, 75
Bicitra. *see* Citric acid, sodium citrate with
Bier block, 78

Billroth I procedure, 16t
Billroth II procedure, 16t
Binaural hearing, definition of, 51t
Bipolar cautery, 40, 50f
Bishop Harmon tissue forceps, 41t–49t
Bladder, procedures for, 109–111
Blepharoplasty (eyelid repair or reconstruction),
 133f
Blunt rake retractors, 41t–49t
Body parts, terms for, 3, 4t
Bolsters, surgical, 67–68
Bookwalter retractors, 41t–49t
Bordetella pertussis, 61
Breast, 20, 20f
 surgeries in, 20–21, 97–98
Breast cancer, surgical management for, 96f
Breast reconstruction, procedures for, 135–136
Bridges, surgical, 67, 68f
Broad-spectrum penicillins, 77
Bronchoscopy, 124
Burns, types of, 131–132

C

Caldwell-Luc antrostomy, 99, 99f
Campylobacter jejuni, 61
Cardiothoracic surgery, perioperative case
 management for, 122–126, 124f
Cardiovascular system
 blood flow in, 138f
 other procedures for, 12
 peripheral, 136–137
 surgeries in, 10–12
Carotid endarterectomy, 27t, 31–32, 32f, 140, 140b,
 140f
Carpal tunnel release, 29, 29t
Castroviejo needle holders, 41t–49t
Cataract, procedures for, 118, 119f, 120b
Cavitron Ultrasonic Surgical Aspirator (CUSA),
 40, 53t
Ceclor. *see* Cefaclor
Cefaclor, 76
Cefadroxil, 76
Cefadryl. *see* Cefapirin
Cefapirin, 76
Cefazolin, 76
Cefepime, 77
Cefixime, 77
Cefizox. *see* Ceftizoxime
Cefmetazole, 76
Cefobid. *see* Cefoperazone
Cefoperazone, 77
Cefotan. *see* Cefotetan
Cefotaxime, 76
Cefotetan, 76
Cefoxitin, 76
Cefprozil, 76
Cefradine, 76
Ceftazidime, 77
Ceftin. *see* Cefuroxime

Note: Page numbers followed by *f* indicate figure, by *t* table, and by *b* box.